AAS
Agents and Actions Supplements
Vol. 31

Series Editor
K. Brune, Erlangen

Birkhäuser Verlag
Basel · Boston · Berlin

Mediators in Airway Hyperreactivity

Edited by

Frans P. Nijkamp
Ferdi Engels
Paul A. J. Henricks
Antoon J. M. Oosterhout

1990

Birkhäuser Verlag
Basel · Boston · Berlin

Volume Editors' Address:

F. P. Nijkamp
F. Engels
P. A. J. Henricks
A. J. M. Van Oosterhout

University of Utrecht
Faculty of Pharmacy
Department of Pharmacology
Catharijnesingel 60
NL–3511 GH Utrecht / The Netherlands

Deutsche Bibliothek Cataloging-in-Publication Data

Mediators in airway hyperreactivity / ed. by Frans P. Nijkamp
... – Basel ; Boston ; Berlin : Birkhäuser, 1990
(Agents and actions : Supplements ; Vol. 31)
ISBN 3-7643-2513-5 (Basel ...) Gb.
ISBN 0-8176-2513-5 (Boston) Gb.
NE: Nijkamp, Frans P. [Hrsg.]; Agents and actions / Supplements

Product Liability: The publisher can give no guarantee for information about drug dosage and application thereof contained in this book. In every individual case the respective user must check its accuracy by consulting other pharmaceutical literature.

Printed in Germany on acid-free paper from the authors' camera-ready manuscripts
ISBN 3-7643-2513-5
ISBN 0-8176-2513-5

CONTENTS

INFLAMMATORY CELLS and MEDIATORS

CYTOKINES

PLATELET-ACTIVATING FACTOR

EPITHELIUM-DERIVED FACTORS

PREFACE AND ACKNOWLEDGEMENT

For more than five decades it has been recognized that the release or generation of a range of mediators accounts for the features of asthma exacerbation. Progressive classification of these chemical structures in the last decade has revealed that these mediators not only control acute bronchoconstriction, but also contribute to the late asthmatic reaction, changes in vascular permeability, mucus secretion and the inflammatory reaction. The number of mediators which play a role in the asthmatic reactions is still extending. Nowadays it is recognized that important (classes of) mediators are the eicosanoids, a number of neuropeptides, platelet activating factor, a number of epithelium derived factors. It has become recently apparent that also the cytokines may play a major role in the modulation of the asthmatic reaction. Besides the direct effects, mediators also contribute to hyperreactivity of the airways to non-specific stimuli, a general feature in more than 80% of the asthmatic patients.

In order to review the fast developments with respect to the role of asthma-mediators in airway hyperreactivity, an international meeting was held in The Hague (Kijkduin), The Netherlands on June 28-30, 1990 to integrate the numerous important advances in our understanding of biochemical, physiological and cellular processes in airway hyperreactivity. To this end, we invited a group of international experts to present an overview of their particular field of research. The overviews were completed with a number of small presentations and posters. The format of the meeting favored extensive discussions.

It is hoped that this volume will be appreciated as a contribution to the better understanding of the role of the different mediators in airway hyperreactivity.

This meeting was made possible by financial support from GLAXO - The Netherlands. This generosity is gratefully acknowledged.

F.P. Nijkamp
F. Engels
P.A.J. Henricks
A.J.M. Van Oosterhout

AAS 31:
Mediators in
Airway Hyperreactivity

AIRWAY HYPERREACTIVITY, AN INTRODUCTION

R. Pauwels, J. Kips and G. Joos

Department of Respiratory Diseases, University Hospital,
De Pintelaan 185, B9000, Ghent, Belgium.

SUMMARY: Asthma is characterized by the presence of airway inflammation and an increased responsiveness to many different stimuli. The hyperresponsiveness to indirect stimuli such as adenosine, bradykinin, neuropeptides, sulphur dioxide suggest that the hyperresponsiveness in asthma results from the complex interaction between inflammatory cells, neurons and smooth muscle cells. Several mechanisms may be involved in the influence of airway inflammation on airway responsiveness: increased mucosa permeability: enhanced exposure of irritant receptors, modulation of airway smooth muscle behavior by inflammatory mediators, mucosal edema, enhanced release of neurotransmitters, increased local reflex activity, decreased breakdown of neurotransmitters, etc. We have investigated the interaction between airway inflammation and responsiveness in two animal models: acute exposure to endotoxin and chronic exposure to aerosolized antigen. Both models demonstrate the complexity of interaction between inflammatory processes and demonstrate positive controlling mechanisms that inhibit the increase in airway responsiveness due to airway inflammation. The lack of such controlling mechanisms may be involved in the development of the asthmatic airway hyperresponsiveness.

An increased responsiveness to various stimuli is an important pathophysiological characteristic of bronchial asthma. The aim of the present paper is to review some of the possible mechanisms involved in the bronchial hyperresponsiveness of asthmatics and to present some of the experimental work that we have performed on the relation between inflammation and airway hyperresponsiveness. We also present the results of pharmacological investigations in the different experimental models.

In asthmatics, acute bronchoconstriction can be provoked by several stimuli including allergens, exercise, cold air, fog, air pollutants, cigarette smoke, the intake of drugs such as aspirin, etc. The mechanisms involved in the acute bronchial response to these triggers are partially understood. The bronchoconstrictor response to different stimuli is mediated via interaction with receptors situated on the bronchial smooth muscle cells, or with receptors on inflammatory cells such as mast cells and macrophages leading to the liberation of mediators that act on the smooth muscle cells or nerve receptors, or by stimulation of the sensory nerve receptors leading to local axon reflexes or vagal-mediated central nervous reflexes. It is easily conceivable that most of the stimuli causing symptoms in asthmatics do not act directly on the bronchial smooth muscle cell (1). The mucosa and the submucosa act as a barrier between the inspired air and the bronchial smooth muscle layer. Damage to the epithelium may cause a better penetration of stimuli in the airway wall. The local axon reflex arises by stimulation of a sensory nerve ending and the antidromical release of one or more transmitters from axon collaterals (2). The transmitters of these axon reflexes are not known but there are reasons to believe that both neuropeptides and adenosine may be involved (3,4). The presence of neuropeptides, such as substance P and neurokinin A, and of nucleosides, more specifically ATP that is rapidly degraded to adenosine upon release, has been demonstrated in neurons of the airways. Neuropeptides including neurokinin A cause bronchoconstriction both in experimental animals and in man (5,6). Adenosine has been shown to cause bronchoconstriction in rats and in asthmatic patients (7,8). There is now evidence that both the neuropeptides and adenosine cause bronchoconstriction by an interaction with specific receptors on vagal nerve endings and mast cells (9). The simultaneous release of acetylcholine from nerve endings and smooth muscle constricting agents from mast cells causes a synergistic bronchoconstriction. We have also observed in the animal model that adenosine and neurokinin A act synergistically in inducing mast cell activation and airway narrowing.

The influence of various pharmacological agents on the bronchoconstriction induced by different non-specific stimuli supports the hypothesis of indirect mechanisms being important in the airway response of asthmatics to different stimuli (Table I)(1). Animal data suggest that cromoglycate and nedocromil inhibit the local axon reflex mechanisms at least partially by inhibition of the release of inflammatory mediators from mast cells. Xanthines inhibit the local axon reflex mechanisms by an as yet not identified mechanism but do not seem to inhibit the activation of mast cells involved in this local axon reflex.

Clinical, epidemiological and experimental data suggest that the bronchial responsiveness is determined both by genetic and exogenous factors (10). In previous investigations we have demonstrated that inbred rat strains differ substantially with regard to their bronchial responsiveness and breeding experiments confirmed the importance of genetic factors influencing the bronchial responsiveness to 5-hydroxytryptamine (11). In vitro experiments have confirmed the presence of strain differences in bronchial smooth muscle responsiveness (12). Family studies and twin studies suggest that also in man genetic factors regulate the airway responsiveness to methacholine and exercise (13,14).

The degree of bronchial responsiveness is not fixed and may increase following an upper respiratory tract infection, after acute or chronic exposure to allergens, following exposure to air pollutants, and during occupational exposure to sensitizing agents. Bronchial hyperresponsiveness has also been shown to decrease by avoidance of the causative allergens or occupational

Table I. Inhibitory effect of drugs on the bronchoconstrictor activity of different stimuli.

DRUG	EXERCISE	OSMOTIC	SO_2	COLD AIR	ADENOSINE	NK A	PROPRANOLOL
Sympathomimetics	++++	+++	+++	+++			
Theophylline	++	++		++	+++		
Anticholinergics	+	++	+++	++	+/-	+/-	+
Steroids	-/+++						
SCG	+++	+++	+++	+++	+++		+++
Nedocromil	+++	+++	+++	+++	+++	+++	
Ketotifen	++	++		++			
H_1-antagonists	++				++		

agents and during treatment with sodium cromoglycate or corticosteroids.

Subacute airway inflammation has been hypothesized to play an important role in the modulation of non specific bronchial responsiveness and in particular neutrophils, eosinophils and platelets have been put forward as cells involved in this process (15,16,17). A striking example of this association between airway inflammation and changes in airway responsiveness is the late reaction following allergen challenge (18).

The mechanisms involved in the changes in airway responsiveness induced by airway inflammation are not yet fully identified. Possible mechanisms involved are:

- increased permeability of the airway epithelium, so that triggering substances can more easily reach their target receptor
- increased sensitivity of irritant receptors
- increased release of neurotransmitters from neurons caused by a change in the activation status of the neurons or a change in the quantity and the quality of the neurotransmitters contained in the neurons or a change in the number of neurons
- increased number of effector cells e.g. mast cells
- decreased metabolism of neurotransmitters or inflammatory mediators
- increased reactivity of airway smooth muscle cells due to an increase in receptors are an enhanced receptor-coupling
- synergism between inflammatory mediators and neurotransmitters
- edema of the airway wall leading to a change in airway mechanics so that for the same degree of airway smooth muscle contraction a much more important airway narrowing is observed. The enhanced airway narrowing in asthmatics may also be related to an uncoupling of the normal elastic recoil pressure. This mechanism could be the explanation

of the absence of a plateau in the dose response-curve to histamine or methacholine in asthmatics.

Clinical studies in asthma suggest that several of these mechanisms are indeed present in asthmatics and it is very improbable that anyone particular mechanism will explain all the abnormalities in airway responsiveness in asthmatics. Both animal studies and clinical studies will help us to understand the mechanisms involved in the clinical disease and to develop new therapeutic strategies.

We therefore decided to study the influence of airway inflammation on bronchial responsiveness in the rat model (19). Airway inflammation was induced by exposing the animals to an aerosol of endotoxin. The exposure to an aerosol of endotoxin caused in F344 rats a rapid influx of neutrophils in the airways The neutrophils persisted up to 24 hours after exposure. The exposure to the endotoxin-aerosol was followed, one to two hours later, by a significant increase in the airway responsiveness to 5-hydroxytryptamine (5HT). However, the increase in responsiveness disappeared and nine to twelve hours following the end of the exposure a significant decrease in airway 5HT-responsiveness was observed at a moment that more than eighty percent of the cells contained in the BAL fluid were neutrophils. Analysis of the elastase concentration in the lavage fluid, as parameter of neutrophil activation, suggests that the presence of activated neutrophils in the airways does not correlate with the increase in responsiveness or that other mediators secreted by these cells are involved in the hyperresponsiveness.

We also compared the effect of endotoxin-inhalation in three different inbred rat strains. The aerosol exposure induced in all three strains a comparable neutrophil influx in the airways but only two of the three strains became hyperresponsive to 5HT. Endotoxin inhalation equally increased the airway responsiveness to carbachol, adenosine and neurokinin A but did not enhance the mast cell activation induced by either adenosine or neurokinin A. The relation between airway inflammation and airway responsiveness in this animal model is dependent on the time following the exposure, the animal strain and the type of agent used for the assessment of airway responsiveness.

We also investigated the effect of anti-asthmatic drugs on the airway inflammation and increase in bronchial responsiveness following endotoxin exposure in the rat model that we have developed. The animals were injected intraperitoneally, 30 minutes before the start of the endotoxin exposure with the following solutions in a volume of 0.5 ml saline, ketotifen 0.1 mg/kg, ketotifen 0.3 mg/kg, ketotifen 1 mg/kg, aminophylline 15 mg/kg, sodium cromoglycate 1 mg/kg, terbutaline 0.05 mg/kg or methylprednisolone 5 mg/kg. The 5HT-airway responsiveness was assessed 90 minutes after the end of the endotoxin-exposure and was followed by a bronchoalveolar lavage. Endotoxin caused a significant decrease in the percentage of macrophages and a significant increase in the percentage of neutrophils in the pooled bronchoalveolar lavage fluid. Endotoxin had no significant influence on the basal Cdyn and R_L before challenge with 5HT. Pretreatment with aminophylline caused a significant increase in the PC25-Cdyn following endotoxin exposure in comparison with the same parameter following saline pretreatment followed by endotoxin exposure. The same treatment had also a significant influence on the cellular composition of the bronchoalveolar fluid following endotoxin exposure. Following aminophylline treatment there were significantly more macrophages and less neutrophils than in the saline treated, endotoxin exposed group. Essentially the same findings were observed after treatment with sodium cromoglycate. Terbutaline significantly inhibited the endotoxin induced increase in airway responsiveness but had no significant effect on the neutrophil influx. Methylprednisolone pretreatment was followed by a significant higher PC25-Cdyn and PC50-R_L in the endotoxin exposed group compared with the saline pretreated endotoxin exposed group. However methylprednisolone pretreatment did not cause a significant change in the cellular composition of the bronchoalveolar fluid. Ketotifen pretreatment had no significant influence on the increase in bronchial responsiveness or on the changes in cellular composition of the bronchoalveolar lavage fluid following endotoxin exposure. This experiment therefore showed that theophylline, sodium cromoglycate, methylprednisolone and terbutaline administered intraperitoneally half an hour before the exposure of inbred rats to an aerosol of endotoxin partially inhibited the increase in bronchial responsiveness to 5HT. Theophylline, sodium cromoglycate and terbutaline also partially inhibited the neutrophilic infiltration of the airways following endotoxin exposure. Ketotifen, at the doses and timing used had no significant protective effect.

Following this initial observation on the effect of theophylline and sodium cromoglycate on airway inflammation and bronchial responsiveness we have now performed dose response studies with theophylline, sodium cromoglycate and nedocromil sodium in the same animal model. F344-rats were exposed to either aerosolized saline or endotoxin for 30 minutes. The animals were pretreated, thirty minutes before the start of the aerosol exposure, with an intraperitoneal injection of either saline or aminophylline 5, 10, 15, 20 or 25 mg/kg. 90 minutes after the end of the aerosol exposure, the bronchial responsiveness to i.v. 5HT was determined and bronchoalveolar lavage (BAL) was performed.

The exposure to endotoxin induced a pronounced neutrophilic infiltration of the airways and an increased airway 5HT-responsiveness. Theophylline significantly inhibited the endotoxin-induced airway inflammation and the increase in 5HT-responsiveness. The mean serum theophylline concentrations, immediately before the assessment of the airway responsiveness were respectively 1.4, 5.6, 10.3, 14.3 and 15.7 mg/l in the endotoxin-exposed group. We conclude that theophylline at therapeutic and even lower concentrations inhibits both the endotoxin-induced airway inflammation and increased airway responsiveness.

Sodium cromoglycate in a dose of 0.2 mM, 2 mM and 20 mM/kg and nedocromil sodium in a dose of 0.2 mM, 2mM and 20 mM/kg were administered intraperitoneally 30 minutes before the exposure to endotoxin. Two control groups were included, one exposed to saline instead of endotoxin, and one group exposed to endotoxin but pretreated with saline at 30 minutes before the endotoxin exposure. Both control groups consisted of twelve animals and each treatment group of nine animals. The pretreatment with either nedocromil or cromoglycate did not prevent the endotoxin-induced airway inflammation and increase in bronchial responsiveness.

The endotoxin-model has several aspects that suggest a poor relationship with human asthma including the predominance of neutrophils in the airway inflammation and the short-lived increase in airway responsiveness. We therefore started the development of another rat model, now with predominantly eosinophilic airway inflammation. BN-rats were at day 0 injected intraperitoneally with either adjuvant alone or antigen and adjuvant. From day 10 on, the animals were daily exposed to an aerosol of antigen, each day during 30 minutes. At day 24, we measured airway responsiveness to 5HT and performed bronchoalveolar lavage. BN-rats, injected intraperitoneally with saline and exposed to saline acted as controls. The chronic exposure to aerosolized antigen induced an increase in the number of eosinophils, neutrophils and lymphocytes in the lavage fluid. Pathological examination of the airways in the antigen-exposed animals showed an eosinophilic bronchiolitis. However, in contrast with our expectations, we consistently found a decrease in airway responsiveness following chronic antigen exposure.

The effect of drugs on long-term changes in airway responsiveness in asthmatics may help us to understand the disease and the mode of action of these compounds. Pollen-sensitive asthmatics show an increase in non specific airway responsiveness during the pollen season (20). This increase in responsiveness can be prevented by treatment with cromoglycate (21), nedocromil (22) or corticosteroids (23).

The acute administration of inhaled sympathomimetics causes a consistent decrease in airway responsiveness to histamine or methacholine (24). The effect is dose-related and the duration of the protective effect is dependent on the type of sympathomimetic drug. Long-term administration of inhaled sympathomimetics does not really modify the airway responsiveness to histamine or methacholine, except for a temporary rebound increase in responsiveness after the acute reduction (25). The acute administration of inhaled anticholinergic agents has very little effect on airway responsiveness (26). A transient increase in responsiveness to methacholine was observed after prolonged treatment with inhaled ipratropium (27).

The protective effect of theophylline on direct stimuli such as histamine and methacholine is limited. Acute studies in mild asthma have shown a limited but significant effect against histamine or methacholine induced bronchoconstriction (27,28). Prolonged treatment failed to modify histamine responsiveness in a group of moderate to severe asthmatics (29).

The acute administration of cromoglycate does not modify the responsiveness to methacholine or histamine. The effect of long-term treatment with cromoglycate on non-specific airway responsiveness to histamine or methacholine is rather controversial. Some studies demonstrate a decrease in airway responsiveness following prolonged treatment with cromoglycate

(30,31), others fail to do so (32,33). Nedocromil has no immediate effect on the responsiveness to methacholine or histamine.

Several studies have demonstrated that prolonged treatment with inhaled steroids significantly reduces the airway responsiveness to histamine and methacholine in asthmatics (34-37). The reduction is dose-dependent and takes several weeks before a maximal effect is observed (38). Inhaled steroids have a more pronounced effect than oral steroids on airway responsiveness for doses that have similar effects on lung function (39). However, most asthmatics fail to reach a normal level of airway responsiveness even after prolonged treatment with high doses of the currently available inhaled steroids.

We obviously need studies in humans relating long-term changes in airway responsiveness with changes in airway inflammation before any final conclusion may be reached with regard to the inflammatory mechanisms involved in the pathogenesis of airway inflammation in asthma. The aim of this paper was to present an overview of the possible mechanisms that are involved. We have indeed the tools to look more closely at these mechanisms both in animal models and in asthmatic patients.

REFERENCES

1. Pauwels, R., Joos, G., Van Der Straeten, M. (1988) Bronchial hyperresponsiveness is not bronchial hyperresponsiveness is not bronchial asthma. Clin. Allergy 18, 317-321.
2. Barnes, P.J. (1986) Neural control of human airways in health and disease. Am. Rev. Respir. Dis. 134, 1289-1314.
3. Pauwels, R. (1987) The role of adenosine in bronchial asthma. Clin. Respir. Physiol. 23, 203-208.
4. Joos, G.F.P., Pauwels, R.A.R., Van Der Straeten, M.E.R.P. (1988) The role of neuropeptides as neurotransmitters of non-adrenergic, non-cholinergic nerves in bronchial asthma. Bull. Eur. Physiopathol. Respir. 23, 619-637.
5. Joos, G.F., Pauwels, R.A., Van Der Straeten, M.E. (1988) The mechanism of tachykinin-induced bronchoconstriction in the rat. Am. Rev. Respir. Dis. 137,1038-1044.

6. Joos, G., Pauwels, R., Van Der Straeten, M. (1987) Effect of inhaled substance P and neurokinin A on the airways of normal and asthmatic subjects. Thorax 42, 779-783.
7. Pauwels, R., Van Der Straeten, M. (1987) An animal model for adenosine-induced bronchoconstriction. Am. Rev. Respir. Dis. 136, 374-378.
8. Cushley, M.J., Tattersfield, A.E., Holgate, S.T. (1984) Adenosine-induced bronchoconstriction in asthma. Am. Rev. Respir. Dis. 129, 380-384.
9. Pauwels, R., Joos, G., Kips, J., Van Der Straeten, M. (1989) Interactions between neurotransmitters and inflammatory cells in the airways. Int. Arch. Allergy Clin. Immunol. 88, 68-69.
10. Nadel, J.A., Pauwels, R., Snashall, P.D. (1987) Bronchial Hyperresponsiveness. Blackwell Sc. Publ., Oxford.
11. Pauwels, R., Van Der Straeten, M., Weyne, J., Bazin, H. (1985) Genetic factors in non-specific bronchial reactivity in rats. Eur. J. Respir. Dis. 66, 98-104.
12. Badier, M., Soler, M., Mallea, M., Delpierre, S., Orehek, J. (1988) Cholinergic responsiveness of respiratory and vascular tissues in two different rat strains. J. Appl. Physiol. 64, 323-328.
13. Townley, R., Bewtra, A. (1983) Airway reactivity to methacholine in asthma family members and twins. In: Provocative Challenge Procedures: Bronchial, Oral, Nasal and Exercise (S.L. Spector, Ed.), CRC Press, Boca Raton, pp. 177-183.
14. Konig, P., Godfrey, S. (1974) Exercise-induced bronchial lability in monozygotic (identical) and dizygotic (nonidentical) twins. J. Allergy Clin. Immunol. 54, 280-287.
15. Nadel, J.A. (1984) Inflammation and asthma. J. Allergy Clin. Immunol. 73, 651-653.
16. Wardlaw, A.J., Kay, A.B. (1987) The role of the eosinophil in the pathogenesis of asthma. Allergy 42, 321-335.
17. Morley, J., Sanjar, S., Page, C.P. (1984) The platelet in asthma. Lancet ii, 1142-1144.
18. O'Byrne, P.M., Dolovich, J., Hargreave, F.E. (1987) Late asthmatic responses. Am. Rev. Respir. Dis. 136, 740-751.
19. Pauwels, R., Kips, J.C., Peleman, R., Van Der Straeten, M. (1990) The effect of endotoxin inhalation on airway responsiveness and cellular influx in rats. Am. Rev. Respir. Dis. 141, 540-545.
20. Boulet, L.P., Cartier, A., Thomson, N.C., Roberts, R.S., Dolovich, J., Hargreave, F.E. (1983) Asthma and increases in non allergic bronchial responsiveness from seasonal pollen exposure. J. Allergy Clin. Immunol. 71, 399-406.
21. Löwhagen, O., Rak, S. (1985) Modification of bronchial hyperreactivity after treatment with sodium cromoglycate during pollen season. J. Allergy Clin. Immunol. 75, 460-467.
22. Altounyan, R.E.C., Cole, M., Lee, T.B. (1986) Effect of nedocromil sodium on changes in bronchial hyperreactivity in non-asthmatic, atopic rhinitic patients during the grass

pollen season. Eur. J. Respir. Dis. 69, (Suppl. 147), 271-273.
23. Sotomayor, H., Badier, M., Vervloet, D., Orehek, J. (1984) Seasonal increase of carbachol airway responsiveness in patients allergic to grass pollen. Am. Rev. Respir. Dis. 130, 56-58.
24. Tattersfield, A.E. (1987) Effect of beta-agonists and anticholinergic drugs on bronchial hyperreactivity. Am. Rev. Respir. Dis. 138, S64-S67.
25. Vathenen, A.S., Knox, A.J., Higgins, B.G., Britton J.R., Tattersfield, A.E. (1988) Rebound increase in bronchial responsiveness after treatment with inhaled terbutaline. Lancet i, 554-557.
26. Newcomb, R., Tashkin, D.P., Hui, K.K., Conolly, M.E., Lee, E., Dauphinee, B. (1985) Rebound hyperresponsiveness to muscarinic stimulation after chronic therapy with an inhaled muscarinic antagonist. Am. Rev. Respir. Dis. 132, 12-15.
27. Cartier, A., Lemaire, I., L'Archeveque, J., Ghezzo, H., Martin, R.R., Malo, J-L. (1986) Theophylline partially inhibits bronchoconstriction caused by inhaled histamine in subjects with asthma. J. Allergy Clin. Immunol. 77, 570-575.
28. Magnussen, H., Reuss, G., Jorres, R. (1987) Theophylline has a dose-related effect on the airway response to inhaled histamine and methacholine in asthmatics. Am. Rev. Respir. Dis. 136, 1163-1167.
29. Dutoit, J., Salome, C.M., Woolcock, A.J. (1987) Inhaled corticosteroids reduce the severity of bronchial hyperresponsiveness in asthma but oral theophylline does not. Am. Rev. Respir. Dis. 136, 1174-1178.
30. Furukawa, C.T., Shapiro, G.G., Bierman, C.W., Kraemer, M.J., Ward, D.J., Pierson, W.E. (1984) A double-blind study comparing the effectiveness of cromolyn sodium and sustained-release theophylline in childhood asthma. Pediatrics 74, 453-459.
31. Petty, T.L., Rollins, D.R., Christopher, K., Good, J.T., Oakley, R. (1989) Cromolyn sodium is effective in adult chronic asthmatics. Am. Rev. Respir. Dis. 139, 694-701.
32. Jenkins, C.J., Breslin, A.B. (1987) Long term study of the effect of sodium cromoglycate on non-specific bronchial hyperresponsiveness. Thorax 42, 664-669.
33. Löwhagen, O., Rak, S. (1985) Bronchial hyperreactivity after treatment with sodium cromoglycate in atopic asthmatics not exposed to relevant allergens. J. Allergy Clin. Immunol. 75, 343-347.
34. Ryan, G., Latimer, K.M., Juniper, E.F., Roberts, R.S., Hargreave, F.E. (1985) Effect of beclomethasone diproprionate on bronchial hyperresponsiveness to histamine in controlled nonsteroid-dependent asthmatics. J. Allergy Clin. Immunol. 75, 25-30.
35. Kraan, J., Koëter, G.H., Van de Mark, Th.W., Sluiter, H.J., De Vries, K. (1985) Changes in bronchial hyperreactivity

induced by 4 weeks of treatment with antiasthmatic drugs in patients with allergic asthma : A comparison between budesonide and terbutaline. J. Allergy Clin. Immunol. 76, 628-636.

36. Henriksen, J.M. (1985) Effect of inhalation of corticosteroids on exercise induced asthma : randomised double blind crossover study of budesonide in asthmatic children. Brit. Med. J. 291, 248-249.
37. Kerrebijn, K.F., Van Essen-Zandvliet, E.E.M., Neijens, H.J. (1987) Effect of long-term treatment with inhaled corticosteroids and beta-agonists on the bronchial responsiveness in children with asthma. J. Allergy Clin. Immunol. 79, 653-659.
38. Kraan, J., Koëter, G.H., Van Der Mark, T.W., Boorsma, M., Kukler, J., Sluiter, H.J., De Vries, K. (1988) Dosage and time effects of inhaled budesonide on bronchial hyperreactivity. Am. Rev. Respir. Dis. 137, 44-48.
39. Jenkins, C.R., Woolcock, A.J. (1988) Effect of prednisone and beclomethasone diproprionate on airway responsiveness in asthma: a comparative study. Thorax 43, 378-384.

AAS 31:
Mediators in
Airway Hyperreactivity

AN ALTERNATIVE POINT OF VIEW ON EXPERIMENTAL LUNG HYPERREACTIVITY

S. Desquand, M. Pretolani, J. Lefort and B.B. Vargaftig

Unité de Pharmacologie cellulaire, Unité Associée Institut Pasteur-INSERM n°285, 25, rue du Dr. Roux, 75015, Paris, France.

SUMMARY: The booster injection of antigen to pre-sensitized guinea-pigs induces lung modifications leading to hyperresponsiveness and to shifts in the profile of the effective drugs. The introduction of the concept of lung inflammation offers new targets for drug discovery.

INTRODUCTION

Acute anaphylactic bronchoconstriction (ABC) in sensitized guinea-pigs is widely used for testing anti-allergic drugs. Pharmacologists become satisfied with their model when ABC is evoked consistently and is suppressed by recognized or newly proposed anti-allergic drugs. Their initial apparent success encourages the permanent use of the same procedure for sensitization and for provocation and differences between laboratories are attributed to "errors" or to "animal variations". By doing so, the pharmacologist behaves to a large extent as someone who uses immunology without applying its concepts. Indeed, as we wish to call the attention upon, different procedures of sensitization determine different physiopathological mechanisms and, as a consequence, lead to the development of models for distinct features of asthma with wanted (or unwanted) characteristics.

The procedures recommended in the litterature for active sensitization of guinea-pigs use an antigen, usually ovalbumin, at amounts varying from 1 mg to 100 mg, delivered by the i.p., i.m., s.c. and i.v. routes or by inhalation. Frequently the antigen is associated to complete or incomplete Freunds' adjuvant or to aluminium hydroxide. In all instances, ABC following the provocation with systemic antigen a few weeks later is accounted essentially by histamine release, largely from the liver (Hahn & Oberdorf, 1950). Similarly, ABC following allergen inhalation is attributable to histamine release, together with peptido-leukotrienes (Daffonchio et al., 1989). Since histamine does not account for human asthma, the guinea-pig model was tailored to meet conditions in which its participation is ruled out, by treating the animals with an anti-histamine, with a cyclooxygenase inhibitor (to prevent the participation of cyclooxygenase metabolites and shift the arachidonate metabolism towards the lipoxygenase pathway) and with propranolol, to enhance the sensitivity of the test by suppressing endogenous ß2-mediated bronchodilatation. Under those conditions, lipoxygenase inhibitors are effective against ABC by aerosolized antigen (Payne et al., 1988; Daffonchio et al., 1989) and thus the histamine and cyclooxygenase-suppressed animal is considered as a model for testing lipoxygenase inhibitors and leukotriene (LT) antagonists. It is nevertheless difficult to solve questions concerning the role of mediators and the mode of action of drugs on basis of such a manipulated model, in which adrenergic ß2-mimetics or drugs directed to neuromodulation cannot be tested, because of adrenergic and prostaglandin suppression.

A few years ago, we demonstrated that platelet-activating factor (PAF) induces BC when injected i.v. to the guinea-pig

(Vargaftig et al., 1980) and Halonen et al. (1980) obtained similar results in the rabbit, leading to the hypothesis that PAF mediates the histamine-independent ABC. This concept was reinforced by the demonstration that inhaled PAF also induces BC, even though this response is blocked by aspirin (Lefort & Vargaftig, 1978), contrary to BC following the i.v. injection and in contrast to the situation in human asthma, where cyclooxygenase inhibitors are notoriously ineffective. The discovery that PAF antagonists suppress ABC in passively sensitized animals (Lagente et al., 1987), supported this hypothesis, but doubts were raised when the same antagonists failed to block ABC in actively sensitized guinea-pigs (Pretolani et al., 1987). This contradiction was clarified on light of *ex vivo* studies, using lungs from guinea-pigs sensitized by different procedures tailored to obtain selective responses, as indicated below.

RESULTS-DISCUSSION

HYPERSENSITIVITY AND HYPERRESPONSIVENESS:

Unspecific hyperresponsiveness is an important characteristic of human asthma and follows antigen challenge in experimental situations (Hargreave et al, 1981; Holzmann, 1982). In order to determine the *in vivo* factors leading from hypersensitivity to hyperresponsiveness, we developed an *ex vivo* model in which isolated lungs were obtained from guinea-pigs sensitized with distinct protocols. It became apparent that lungs from actively sensitized and boosted guinea-pigs respond differently to arachidonate and to the inflammatory mediators LTD_4 and particularly PAF (Pretolani et al., 1988), since they undergo an enhanced bronchoconstriction, release larger amounts of thromboxane (Tx) B_2 and are turned into histamine-releasing tissues, as compared to lungs from non-immunized or passively sensitized guinea-pigs. The lung ability to secrete histamine and to form TxB_2 following an intra-arterial injection of 1 ng of PAF increased time-dependently 2, 4 or 7 days after the booster injection of the antigen, showed the same profile as the increase in the capacity of the serum of those guinea-pigs to sensitize tissues from other non-sensitized animals until day 42. Nevertheless, at this time, lung hypersensitivity, i.e., its ability to respond to antigen with ABC and release of mediators as well as the capacity of serum to sensitize isolated tissues had returned to very low levels whereas hyperreactivity persisted for around 3 months (Pretolani et al., 1988). Accordingly, the lung responses to antigen challenge and pulmonary hyperresponsiveness are two distinct events. In those studies, animals had been sensitized twice, a booster injection of antigen being performed 14 days after the first sensitizing injection. Noteworthy was that single-sensitized animals (without the booster), which had low titers of sensitizing specific immunoglobulins, developed hypersensitivity, since their perfused lungs responded to antigen with ABC and release of mediators, but failed to show hyperresponsiveness. The difference between single-sensitized and double-sensitized animals (in both cases, by an active procedure) indicated that the booster injection induces a shift in the lung behaviour. Our present concept is that the booster behaves as a micro-shock which modifies the lung reactivity and provokes a lung disease.

How can the booster injection trigger such a disease? It is clear that a single-sensitized animal should recognize antigen at day 14 when the booster injection is performed, despite the presence of low levels of circulating immunoglobulins. Indeed, at this time, antigen has since long been processed by antigen-presenting cells, the orchestration of T lymphocytes is fully operative and target cells are sensitized. It is thus not surprising that a clinically inapparent micro-shock may follow the booster and thus behave as a mild provocation, resulting in the formation of cytokines which chemoattract and prime inflammatory cells, including neutrophils and eosinophils, for their activation by LTB_4 or PAF. At this stage, we are searching for markers of inflammation to corroborate this hypothesis.

Indirect evidence that hyperresponsiveness following the booster/micro-shock involves an alteration of the behaviour of inflammatory cells was provided by the work of Boukili et al. (1989) who showed that the secretagogue N-formyl-L-methionyl-L-leucyl-L-phenylalanine (FMLP) induces BC and release of TxB_2 when injected at ng amounts into isolated lungs from non-immunized guinea-pigs. As PAF, FMLP failed to trigger the release of histamine from those lungs, but did so when lungs were obtained from actively sensitized and boosted guinea-pigs, TxB_2 being released by lower doses of FMLP as well. In addition, LTB_4 was released by FMLP from the sensitized lungs, even though no such release occured from non-sensitized tissues. Release of LTB_4 by FMLP- and antigen-stimulated lungs from boosted guinea-pigs supports the involvement of leucocytes in our *ex vivo* model of hyperresponsiveness, particularly since the enhanced effects of FMLP were abrogated when the animals were treated with vinblastine after hyperresponsiveness had been established (Boukili et al., submitted). Since vinblastine is known to exhaust circulating granulocytes by depressing haematopoiesis and to interact with the cytoskeleton of granulocytes, it is well possible that it prevents directly the release of histamine by a selected granulocyte-related target, as described for cyclosporin A (Hultsch et al., 1990). The existence of such a target is supported by the fact that a single injection of low doses (10-100 mg/kg) of the anti-allergic drug azelastine to the sensitized guinea-pigs the day of the lung experiment, under *ex vivo* conditions in which its recognized anti-histamine activity is minimized, suppressed selectively the increased PAF-induced release of histamine from the isolated lung, without interfering whatsoever with its effects on non-sensitized lungs (Pretolani et al., submitted). These observations lead to the hypothesis that new target(s) develop in the lung, involving migration, priming or *in situ* differentiation of inflammatory cells after the booster injection of antigen. Our present hypothesis is that in all instances, cytokines are likely to be involved, bridging the gap between lipid and peptide mediation.

DRUG MODULATION OF HYPERRESPONSIVENESS:

Surprisingly, *ex vivo* hyperresponsiveness persisted for at least 3 months, even after the antibody titers and the lung responses to the antigen decreased markedly (Pretolani et al., 1988). Under those conditions, it became possible to study the ability of anti-asthma drugs to interfere with the development of hyperresponsiveness, as a property distinct from the so-called "stabilizing effect", i.e., inhibition of the release of mediators from rat peritoneal populations enriched in mast cells. Modulation of the establishment of hyperresponsiveness should be possible by administering a drug just before the booster injection and for 5-6 days thereafter, until the final *ex vivo* challenge. The test drug was nedocromil sodium which, administered from day 14 to day 20 of the sensitization period, prevented the development of hyperresponsiveness to PAF, both with respect to BC and to the enhanced release of LTC_4 and histamine (Pretolani et al., 1990). At the same time, antigen-induced release of histamine was halved. When nedocromil sodium was infused directly into the isolated lungs, at a concentration of 0.1 mM, no suppression of lung activation was noted, indicating that indeed nedocromil sodium interfered with the development of hyperresponsiveness and not with its expression, as azelastine seems to do. In the course of those experiments, the interesting observation was made that the enrichment in eosinophils of the bronchoalveolar lavage fluid (BAL), triggered by the booster injection, was also suppressed.

HYPERRESPONSIVENESS AND INFLAMMATORY CELLS: HYPOTHETIC MECHANISMS OF RECRUITMENT:

Anti-asthmatic drugs may thus interfere with the inflammatory component of allergic reactions, i.e., migration and/or activation of inflammatory cells, particularly the eosinophils. These cells are found in the BAL of asthmatic patients (Wardlaw et al., 1988) and in the bronchial sub-mucosa of guinea-pigs after ABC or PAF administration (Lellouch-Tubiana et al., 1988). The mechanisms of chemotaxis of the eosinophils are not fully recognized, and it is likely that upon allergen activation resident lung cells, lymphocytes in conjunction with alveolar macrophages, secrete products (monokines? PAF? lipoxygenase derivatives?) which are chemoattractant for eosinophils and/or enhance the expression of adhesive proteins on the endothelium or respiratory epithelium (Wegner et al., 1990). Eosinophils, once activated, release basic proteins toxic for the respiratory epithelium (Frigas et al., 1986). Even though there is also strong evidence for the participation of PAF and of lipoxygenase products of arachidonic acid, the exact role of these derivatives, and particularly their interactions with the cytokines, are unclear presently. In a recent manuscript, Wegner et al. (1990) demonstrated that PAF-exposed eosinophils adhere to endothelial cells where adhesive proteins are induced by endotoxin. This important finding helps to understand how the connection can be made between lipid mediators such as PAF, which appears and acts rapidly, and cytokines, such as those induced by endotoxin, which promote cell adhesion and prime for enhanced secretion and activation upon cell exposure to sub-threshold concentrations of other mediators. The subject was recently reviewed by Zimmermann et al. (1990).

PHARMACOLOGICAL CONSEQUENCES OF THE BOOSTER INJECTION: *EX VIVO* EXPRESSION OF HYPERRESPONSIVENESS:

By definition, PAF antagonists are substances which antagonize PAF. They are usually discovered using platelet aggregation tests and their *in vivo* effectiveness is studied against PAF-induced BC. Since this effect of i.v. PAF is platelet-dependent (Vargaftig et al., 1980), it is not surprising that all PAF antagonists screened on platelets are effective in the guinea-pig BC test. In addition, these antagonists also block BC following the intra-tracheal administration of PAF *in vivo* and BC and release of TxB_2 from isolated platelet-free lungs from non-sensitized guinea-pigs. We were surprised to find that the very same PAF antagonists, which are effective against PAF on non-sensitized lungs, loss their effectiveness against BC and release of TxB_2, histamine and LTC_4, when tested against PAF on lungs from sensitized and boosted animals (Pretolani et al., 1989 a, b). To some extent, this finding suggested that PAF antagonists might be useful to antagonize the effects of a mediator of asthma, PAF, when tested on non-asthmatic animals, some sort of a paradox, as if an anti-asthma agent would be designed to treat... non-asthmatic individuals! Nevertheless, since the increased lung permeability following PAF administration to the lungs was suppressed by the tested antagonists, irrespective of the immune status of the donor animal (Pretolani et al., 1989 b), it became clear that the ability to antagonize PAF on resident cells, such as the endothelium which accounts for the permeability enhancement, was maintained. At this stage, we consider that the booster injection, by modifying the lung behaviour, determines a shift from a PAF-dependent, to a leukotriene-dependent phase, because priming and/or invasion/differentiation leads to a modification of the PAF receptors involved.

PHARMACOLOGICAL CONSEQUENCES OF THE BOOSTER INJECTION: *IN VIVO* EXPRESSION OF HYPERRESPONSIVENESS:

If, as we consider, the *ex vivo* model described above is relevant, an *in vivo* counterpart in the intact animal should be searched for. *In vivo* differences between non-boosted and boosted sensitized animals were indeed identified, but they are rather subtle. In parallel to the *ex vivo* experiments, we found that BC following the intra-tracheal administration of PAF *in vivo*, which is suppressed by aspirin in non-sensitized animals (Lefort & Vargaftig, 1978) becomes refractory to cyclooxygenase inhibition (Desquand et al., 1990 a). In addition, boosted guinea-pigs show an increased permeability of their bronchial epithelium to proteins *in vivo* (Bureau et al., in preparation) and have their BAL enriched in eosinophils (Pretolani et al., 1990). Antigen provocation augments this content, but in higher proportions in boosted, as compared to non-boosted guinea-pigs (Desquand et al., 1990 a). There is no evidence as yet that the eosinophils found in excess in the BAL are activated, but Hirata et al. (1989) demonstrated that, contrary to peritoneal cells, eosinophils from the BAL respond to FMLP; this indicates that after crossing the endothelium and the epithelium, these cells are primed and most likely express receptors otherwise absent from their systemic counterparts.

An important difference between non-boosted and boosted animals was found by Desquand et al. (1990 b). Thus, the PAF antagonist WEB 2086, which had been described as effective against ABC of passively sensitized (Pretolani et al., 1987) and is inactive in our hands against ABC of actively sensitized guinea-pigs, did suppress ABC on actively sensitized animals for 2-4 days after the booster, and loss its effectiveness later, confirming the concept that the booster injection determines a radical modification of the behaviour of the bronchopulmonary responses of the guinea-pig.

Other markers for the difference between boosted and non-boosted animals have been located by Bachelet et al. (1989) in the alveolar macrophage. This cell builds up its content of cyclic AMP when exposed to prostaglandin E_2 or to the ß-adrenergic agonist salbutamol, but this enhancement was markedly reduced when the cells were obtainted from the BAL of boosted animals, as if their capacity to auto-restrain activation via cyclic AMP increment had been reduced during sensitization (Brunelleschi et al., 1990).

CONCLUSION: Models for asthma have two requirements: they should allow appropriate analyses of the mechanisms involved and of the potential sites of action of drugs and should fit to the human situation. Our *ex vivo* model allows the study of the lung-born mediators, of the role of resident and invasive cells and of the *in situ* and *ex vivo* modulation with drugs. In addition, since hypersensitivity and hyperresponsiveness were dissociated in time and pharmacologically, the model clearly fits to the human situation, in which a patient is continuously exposed to an allergen, thus perpetuating the recruitment and activation of inflammatory cells. The pertinence of the *in vitro* findings was extended *in vivo*, since aspirin and PAF antagonists showed modified properties, according to the boosted or non-boosted status of the animal used. Of course, many questions remain unanswered: which is the cellular and molecular basis for the booster-induced trigger? Are interleukins and neuropeptides involved, leading to in situ priming and/or activation? These and other questions should be answered in the near future.

REFERENCES

Bachelet, M., Masliah, J., Malanchère, E., Lefort, J., Béréziat, G., and Vargaftig, B.B. (1989) Reduced responsiveness of bronchoalveolar cells from sensitised guinea-pigs to the cyclic AMP-stimulating effect of prostaglandin E_2 and ß-adrenoceptor agonists, Pulmonary Pharmacol. 2, 41-44.

Boukili, M.A., Bureau, M., Lellouch-Tubiana, A., Lefort, J., Simon, M.T., and Vargaftig, B.B. (1989) Alveolar macrophages and eicosanoids, but not neutrophils, mediate bronchoconstriction induced by fMLP in the guinea-pig, Br. J. Pharmacol. 98, 61-70.

Brunelleschi, S., Vanni, L., and Fantozzi, R. (1990) Sensory neuropeptides activate guinea-pig alveolar macrophages, Eur. J. Pharmacol. 183, 1572.

Daffonchio, L., Lees, I.W., Payne, A.N., and Whittle, B.J.R. (1989) Pharmacological modulation of bronchial anaphylaxis induced by aerosol challenge in anaesthetized guinea-pigs, Br. J. Pharmacol. 9, 701-708.

Desquand, S., Lefort, J., and Vargaftig, B.B. (1990 a) The booster injection of antigen turns aspirin inactive against bronchoconstriction by intratracheal PAF and increases the pulmonary recruitment of eosinophils by antigen and PAF, J. Lipid Med. 32, 193.

Desquand, S., Lefort, J., Dumarey, C., and Vargaftig, B.B. (1990 b) The booster injection during active guinea-pig sensitisation modulates the anti-anaphylactic activity of the PAF antagonist compound WEB 2086, Br. J. Pharmacol. 100, 217-222.

Frigas, E., and Gleich, G.J. (1986) The eosinophil and the pathophysiology of asthma, J. Allergy Clin. Immunol. 77, 527-537.

Hahn, F., and Oberdorf, A. (1950) Antihistaminica und anaphylaktoide reaktionen, Z. Immunitaetforsch Exp. Ther. 107, 528.

Halonen, M., Palmer, J.D., Lohman, I.C., McManus, L.M., and Pinckard, R.N. (1980) Respiratory and circulatory alterations induced by acetyl glyceryl ether phosphorylcholine (AGEPC), a mediator of IgE anaphylaxis in the rabbit, Am. Rev. Respir. Dis. 122 915-924.

Hargreave, F.E., Ryan, G., Thomson, N.C. O'Byrne, P.M., Latiner, K., Juniper, E.F. and Dolovich, J. (1981) Bronchial responsiveness to histamine or methacholine in asthma: measurement and clinical significance, J. Allergy Clin. Immunol. 68, 347-355.

Hirata, K., Pelé, J.P., Robidoux, C., and Sirois, P. (1989) Guinea-pig lung eosinophil: purification and prostaglandin production, J. Leuko. Biol. 45, 523-528.

Holzmann, N.J. (1982) Pathophysiology of asthma: an overview of mechanisms of bronchial hyperreactivity. In: Bronchial hyperreactivity (J. Morley, Ed) Academic Press/London, pp. 5-17.

Hultsch, T., Rodriguez, J.L., Kaliner, M.A., and Hohman, R.J. (1990) Cyclosporin A inhibits degranulation of rat basophil leukemia cells and human basophils, J. Immunol. 144, 2659-2664.

Lagente, V., Touvay, C., Randon, J., Desquand, S., Cirino, M., Vilain, B., Lefort, J., Braquet, P., and Vargaftig, B.B. (1987) Interference of Paf-acether antagonist BN 52021 with passive anaphylaxis in the guinea-pig, Prostaglandins 33, 265-274.

Lefort, J., and Vargaftig, B.B. (1978) Role of platelets in aspirin-sensitive BC in the guinea-pig; interactions with salicylic acid, Br. J. Pharmacol. 63, 35-42.

Lellouch-Tubiana, A., Lefort, J., Simon, M.T., Pfister, A., and Vargaftig, B.B. (1988) Eosinophil recruitment into guinea pig lungs after PAF-acether and allergen administration. Modulation by prostacyclin, platelet depletion, and selective antagonists, Am. Rev. Respir. Dis. 137, 948-954.

Payne, A.N., Garlard, L.G., Lees, I.W., and Salmon, J.A. (1988) Selective inhibition of arachidonate 5-lipoxygenase by novel acetohydroxamic acids: effects on bronchial anaphylaxis in anaesthetized guinea-pigs, Br. J. Pharmacol. 94, 540-546.

Pretolani, M., Lefort, J., Malanchère, E., and Vargaftig, B.B. (1987) Interference of the novel PAF-acether antagonist WEB 2086 with the bronchopulmonary responses to PAF-acether and to active and passive shock in the guinea-pig, Eur. J. Parmacol. 140, 311-321.

Pretolani, M., Lefort, J., and Vargaftig, B.B. (1988) Active immunization induces lung hyperresponsiveness in the guinea pig. Pharmacological modulation and triggering role of the booster injection, Am. Rev. Respir. Dis. 138, 1572-1578.

Pretolani, M., Lefort, J., Dumarey, C., and Vargaftig, B.B. (1989 a) Role of lipoxygenase metabolites for the hyper-responsiveness to platelet-activating factor of lungs from actively sensitized guinea pigs, J. Pharmacol. Exp. Ther. 248, 353-359.

Pretolani, M., Lefort, J., and Vargaftig, B.B. (1989 b) Limited interference of specific Paf antagonists with hyperresponsiveness to PAF itself of lungs from actively sensitized guinea-pigs, Br. J. Pharmacol. 97, 433-442.

Pretolani, M., Lefort, J., Silva, P., Malanchère, E., Dumarey, C., Bachelet, M., and Vargaftig, B.B. (1990) Protection by nedocromil sodium of active immunization-induced broncho-pulmonary alterations in the guinea-pig, Am. Rev. Respir. Dis. 141, 1259-1265.

Vargaftig, B.B., Lefort, J., Chignard, M., Benveniste, J. (1980) Platelet-activating factor induces a platelet-dependent bronchoconstriction unrelated to the formation of prostaglandin derivates, Eur. J. Pharmacol. 65, 185-192.

Wardlaw, A.J., Dunnette, S., Gleich, G.J., Collins, J.V., and Kay, A.B. (1988) Eosinophils and mast cells in bronchoalveolar lavage in subjects with mild asthma, Am. Rev. Respir. Dis. 137, 62-70.

Wegner, C.D., Gunder, R.H., Reilly, P., Haynes, N., Letts, L.G., and Rothlein, R. (1990) Intercellular adhesion molecule-1 (ICAM-1) in the pathogenesis of asthma, Science 247, 456-459.

Zimmermann, G.A., McIntyre, T.M., Prescott, S.M., and Otsuka, K. (1990) Brief review: molecular mechanisms of neutrophils binding to endothelium involving platelet-activating factor and cytokines, J. Lipid. Med. 2, 531-543.

AAS 31:
Mediators in
Airway Hyperreactivity

ISOLATED AND DUAL TYPE OF LATE ASTHMATIC RESPONSE (LAR) - THE CLINICAL CHARACTERISTICS AND PHARMACOLOGIC CONTROL

Z. Pelikan and M. Pelikan-Filipek

Dept. of Allergology & Immunology, Inst. Med. Sci. "De Klokkenberg", Galderseweg 81, Breda, The Netherlands

INTRODUCTION

The purpose of this study was to investigate: (1) the frequency of the late asthmatic response (LAR) to allergen challenge and its two modifications, the isolated late asthmatic response (ILAR) and the dual late asthmatic response (DLAR); (2) the association of both the modifications of LAR with other "in vivo" and "in vitro" diagnostic parameters; (3) the protective effects of various drugs on the LAR and its two modifications.

In 122 patients suffering from allergic bronchial asthma, besides a routine diagnostic procedure, 353 bronchial challenges (BPT) with various inhalant allergens were also performed using spirography.

The VC (vital capacity) and FEV_1 (forced expiratory 1-second volume) values were recorded up to 56 hours after the allergen challenge. The FEV_1 values were considered to be the basic parameters for the assessment of the bronchial obstruction.

In each of the patients studied a control challenge with PBS (Phosphate Buffered Saline) was also performed and recorded up to 56 hours. In these patients various "in vitro" and "in vivo" diagnostic parameters were also recorded (intracutaneous tests, total and specific IgE in the serum, total IgG, IgM, IgA in the serum, eosinophil and leucocyte count in the blood, body temperature, bronchial and general complaints, leucocyte histamine releasing test, bronchial threshold for histamine, in some of the patients also for metacholine).

In patients developing positive asthmatic responses, protection tests with various drugs were performed. The pre-treatment with the appropriate drug was always started 60 hours before and continued up to 56 hours after the allergen challenge.

In all positive cases of the isolated immediate asthmatic responses (IAR; n = 134), isolated late (ILAR; n = 57) and dual late response (DLAR; n = 60), the protection tests with disodium cromoglycate (DSCG; in a daily dose of 4 x 1 capsule containing 20 mg DSCG powder by spinhaler), Beclomethasone dipropionate or Budesonide (BDA, n = 121; BSA, n = 130; both of them in a daily dose of 4 x 200 mcg inhaled from a pressurized container), and Salbutamol (SBT; in a daily dose of 4 x 200 mcg powder inhaled from a special inhaler) were carried out.

In some cases additional protection tests with other drugs were performed, with Thiazinamium methyl-sulphate (THM; n = 12 IAR, 16 LAR; in a daily dose of 3 x 200 mg orally), Theophylline (TPA; n = 10 IAR, 15 LAR; in a dialy dose of 2 x 350 mg retard orally), Promethazine hydrochloride (PMH; n = 8 IAR, 8 LAR; in a daily dose of 3 x 10 mg orally), Isoprenaline (IPS; n = 7 IAR, 8 LAR; in a daily dose of 3 x 8 inhalations of 0,1 % dilution in distilled water) and Nedocromil sodium aerosol (NDS; n = 12 IAR, 25 LAR; in a daily dose of 4 x 4 mg inhaled from a pressurized container).

RESULTS

(1) Of the 353 bronchial challenges performed in 122 patients, 102 negative bronchial responses (= 29 %) ($p > 0.1$)

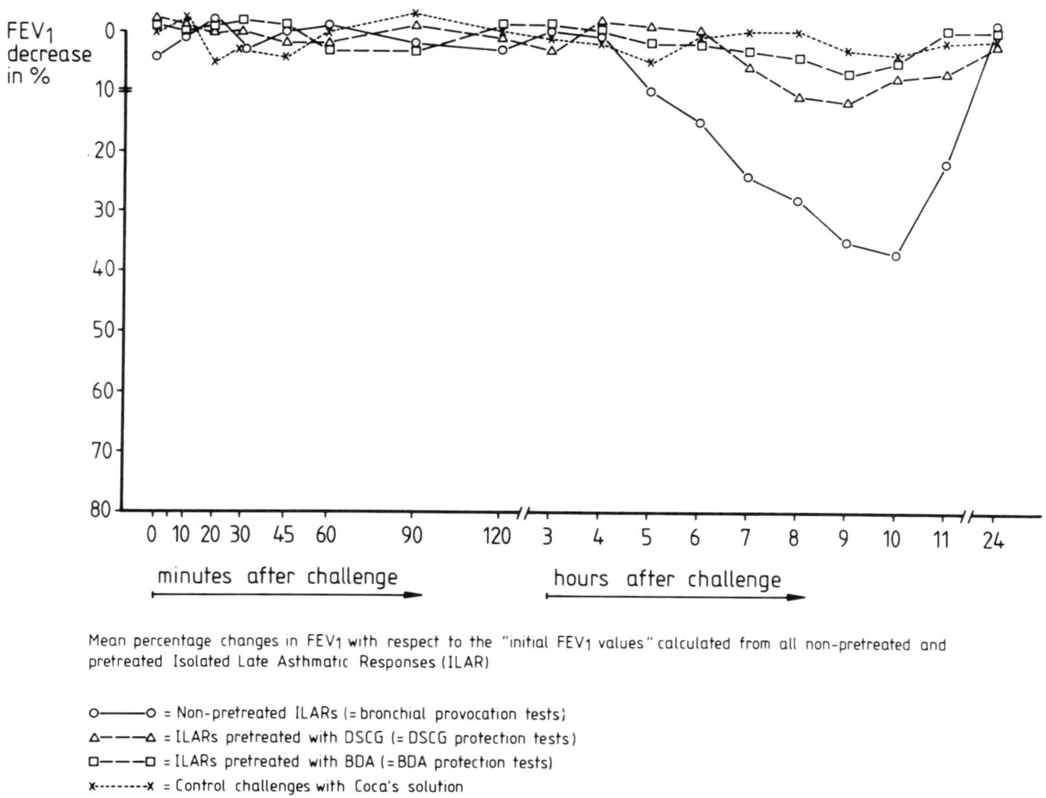

Fig. 1. Effects of disodium chromoglycate and beclomethasone dipropionate on the late asthmatic response to allergen challenge.

and 251 positive asthmatic responses (= 71 %) ($p < 0.05$) were recorded.

(2) Of the 251 positive responses, 134 isolated immediate responses (IAR; = 38 %) and 117 late responses (LAR; = 33 %) were recorded.

Two types of the late response were recorded: 57 cases of isolated late response (ILAR; = 16 %) (Fig. 1) and 60 cases of dual late response (DLAR; = 17 %), which is a combination of an immediate (IDAR) and a late (LDAR) response (Fig. 2).

(3) The IAR began within 10, reached its maximum within 45, and resolved within 120 minutes [2,5], while the LAR began within 4-6, reached its maximum within 12 and resolved within 26 hours after the allergen challenge [1,3,4,6].

(4) The association of the IAR and both the modification of the LAR with other diagnostic parameters is presented in Table I, while the bronchial and general complaints accompanying the particular types of asthmatic response are reviewed in Table II.

(5) Of the 122 patients, 31 demonstrated decreased bronchial threshold to histamine, while 91 did not. Of the 43 patients, 9 developed a decreased bronchial treshold to metacholine.

(6) The blood cell count showed a relative increase in eosinophils and neutrophils, with a slight shifting to the left and an increase in the platelet count within 30-120 minutes before the onset of LAR in 89 cases.

(7) The ILAR was prevented highly by BDA/BSA, DSCG and NDS, slightly by SBT and TPA, while THM, PMH and IPS were ineffective. The DLAR was prevented highly by DSCG, NDS and BDA/BSA, partially by SBT and TPA, while THM, PMH and IPS were ineffective. In contrast, the IAR was prevented highly by DSCG, partially by SBT, THM and NDS, slightly by TPA and IPS, while PMH and BDA/BSA were ineffective (Table III).

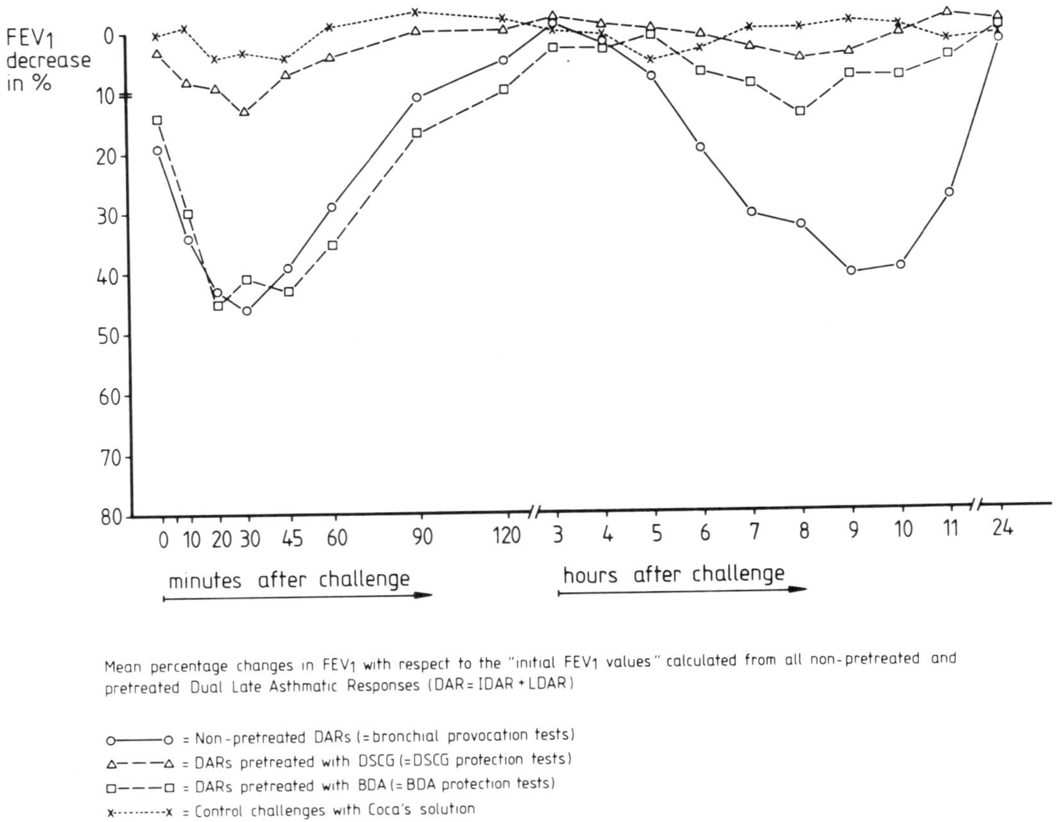

Fig. 2. Effects of disodium chromoglycate and beclomethasone dipropionate on the late asthmatic response to allergen challenge.

Table I
Results of other diagnostic parameters

		BRONCHIAL RESPONSE			
		positive late n = 117			
		dual n = 60	isolated n = 57	immmediate n = 134	negative n = 102
POSITIVE SKIN RESPONSE	Immediate	35	11	98	57
	Late	33	43	16	3
INCREASE IN TOTAL IgE in the serum (RIST)		7	1	41	4
POSITIVE SPECIFIC IgE in the serum (RAST)		11	0	55	8
INCREASE IN IgG in the serum		40	42	34	5
INCREASE IN IgM in the serum		8	13	3	1
INCREASE IN IgA in the serum		1	0	0	1
INCREASE IN BLOOD EOSINOPHILS/ LEUCOCYTES		20/7	31/13	27/20	5/6
INCREASE IN BODY TEMPERATURE		3	8	0	0
EARLY BRONCHIAL COMPLAINTS		60	0	134	0
LATE BRONCHIAL COMPLAINTS		60	57	0	0
LATE GENERAL MALAISE		7	15	0	0
LEUCOCYTE HISTAMINE RELEASE TEST-POSITIVE		24	9	35	1

Table II
Review of the bronchial and general complaints accompanying the immediate and late bronchial response

	Response	
	Immediate	Late
Dyspnea	++	+++
Wheezing	+++	+
Cough	+++	±
Expectoration		
- thick sputum	-	+
- thin sputum	++	-
Pressure on the chest	-	+
Chills	-	+
Tiredness	-	+
Headache	-	++
Weakness	-	+++

Table III
Protective effects of the drugs tested

Drug	IMMEDIATE ASTHMATIC RESPONSE	LATE ASTHMATIC RESPONSE	
		ISOLATED	PART OF DUAL
Disodium cromoglycate	++++	++	+++
Beclomethason diprop./ Budesonide	-	+++	++
Thiazinamium methyl-sulfate	+±	-	±
Salbutamol	++	+	+±
Theophylline	+	+	+±
Promethazine hydrochl.	-	-	-
Isoprenaline	+	-	-
Nedocromil Sodium*	+±	++±	++

* Supplementary results in 12 IAR, 10 ISOLATED "LAR", 15 DUAL "LAR"

CONCLUSIONS

The late asthmatic response is associated with other diagnostic parameters to different degrees than the immediate asthmatic response [2-4]. Their pharmacologic modulation and control by individual basic drugs also demonstrate distinct differences [1-6]. The exact mechanism underlying the late asthmatic response and both its sub-types is not yet fully known [3,4,6].

However, this study, demonstrating not only the differences in the clinical course and in the association with other diagnostic parameters, but also the differences in the pharmacologic modulation of the IAR and both the sub-types of LAR by individual drugs, might suggest the possible involvement of different hypersensitivity mechanisms in them. The involvement of late hypersensitivity in the late asthmatic response could be presumed to be one of the possible mechanisms [3,6].

REFERENCES

[1] Cockcroft, D.W., Murdock, K.Y. (1987) Protective effect of inhaled albuterol, cromolyn, beclomethasone and placebo on allergen-induced early asthmatic responses, late asthmatic responses and allergen-induced increases in bronchial responsiveness to inhaled histamine. J. Allergy Clin. Immunol. 79, 734.

[2] Pelikan, Z., Pelikan-Filipek, M., Kruis, M., and Berger, M.P.F. (1986) The immediate asthmatic response to allergen challenge. Annals of Allergy, 56, 252-260.

[3] Pelikan, Z., and Pelikan-Filipek M. (1986) The late asthmatic response to late allergen challenge, Part I + II. Annals of Allergy, 56, 414-420, 421-435.

[4] Pelikan, Z., Schot, J.D.L., and Koedijk, F.H.J. (1983) The late bronchus-obstructive response to bronchial challenge with pigeon feaces and its correlation with precipitating antibodies (IgG) in the serum of patients having long-term contact with pigeons. Clin. Allergy, 13, 203-211.

[5] Pelikan, Z., Pelikan-Filipek, M., Schoemaker, C., and Berger, M.P.F. (1988) Effects of disodium cromoglycate and beclomethasone dipropionate on the asthmatic response to allergen challenge. I. Immediate Response (IAR). Annals of Allergy, 60, 211-216.

[6] Pelikan, Z., Pelikan-Filipek, M., and Remeijer, L. (1988) Effects of disodium cromoglycate and beclomethasone dipropionate on the asthmatic response to allergen challenge. II. Late Response (LAR). Annals of Allergy, 60, 217-225.

AAS 31:
Mediators in
Airway Hyperreactivity

DELAYED ASTHMATIC RESPONSE (DAR) AND ITS PHARMACOLOGIC MODULATION

Z. Pelikan

Dept. of Allergology & Immunology, Inst. Med. Sci. "De Klokkenberg", Galderseweg 81, Breda, The Netherlands

INTRODUCTION

The purpose of this study was to investigate: (1) the delayed asthmatic response (DAR) to allergen challenge, its clinical feature and association with other "in vivo" and "in vitro" diagnostic parameters; and (2) the possible protective effects of various basic drugs on the "DAR".

In patients with allergic bronchial asthma (BA), besides a routine diagnostic procedure, bronchial challenges with various inhalant allergens (BPT) were also performed. The BPT were performed using spirography. The VC (vital capacity) and FEV_1 (forced expiratory 1-second volume) values were recorded up to 56 hours, if necessary up to 96 hours, after the allergen challenge. The FEV_1 values were considered to be basic parameters for the assessment of the bronchial obstruction.

In each of the patients a control challenge with PBS (Phosphate Buffered Saline) was also performed in the same way as that with allergens. The bronchial response was evaluated according to the following criteria: (a) decrease of FEV_1 or both FEV_1 and VC less than 10% with respect to the PBS control as negative, from 10% to 20% as doubtful, and of 20% or more (PD_{20}) as positive; (b) decrease in FEV_1 values recorded at at least 3 consecutive time intervals, was considered to be positive asthmatic response [1,2].

In 53 of 307 patients suffering from allergic bronchial asthma and having been examined at our department during 1986-1987, an unusual asthmatic response to challenge with various inhalant allergens was recorded. This response, called by us a "delayed asthmatic response" (DAR), became a subject of this study [3].

STUDY DESIGN

In all patients developing the "delayed asthmatic response" (DAR), the bronchial challenge with the same allergen was repeated 1-2 weeks later and supplemented by recording of following "in vivo" and "in vitro" parameters;

(I) Single recording: (a) Intracutaneous tests, recorded at 20 minutes and 8,24,48,96 hours after the allergen injection; (b) Bronchial responsiveness to histamine (PD_{20}).

(II) Multiple recording (before and repeatedly during DAR): (c) IgE total and specific in the serum (PRIST, RAST); (d) IgG, IgM, IgA and subclasses of IgG in the serum; (e) Eosinophil, total leucocyte and leucocyte differential count in the peripheral blood; (f) Histamine in the blood, determined by automated histamine assay in whole blood, according to Siriganian (the histamine [ng/ml] was measured in "blanks"-samples, without any "in vitro" incubation with allergen) [4]; (g) Body temperature; (h) Bronchial complaints, and general malaise complaints.

In the patients developing the "delayed asthmatic response" (DAR), the possible protective effects of various basic drugs on the DAR were also studied. The pre-treatment with the appropriate drug was always started 72 hours before and continued at least up to 56 hours, in some cases to 96 hours, after the allergen challenge.

The following drugs, all of them in the form of a pressurized aerosol, were tested: (a) Disodium cromoglycate (DSCG) - daily dose of 4 x 2 mg; (b) Nedocromil Sodium (NDS)- daily dose of 4 x 4 mg; (c) Salbutamol (SBT) - daily dose of 4 x 400 mcg; (d) Beclomethasone dipropionate (BDA) - daily dose of 4 x 200 mcg; (e) Budesonide (BSA) - daily dose of 4 x 200 mcg.

In each of the patients 3 protection tests were performed; (1) Disodium cromoglycate or Nedocromil; (2) Salbutamol; (3) Beclomethasone or Budesonide. The design of the protection tests was double-blind cross-over. The results were statistically analyzed by Wilcoxon pairs signed ranks' test. (A P value < 0.05 was considered to be statistically significant).

RESULTS

(1) Of the 307 patients with BA, 53 (= 17%) developed so-called "Delayed asthmatic response" (DAR) to allergen challenge ($p < 0.001$). In 52 of the 53 patients the DAR was confirmed by a repeated bronchial challenge.

(2) The "Delayed asthmatic response" (DAR) began within 24-30 hours, reached its maximum within 30-48 hours, and resolved within 56, sometimes 96 hours (Fig. 1).

(3) The DAR was accompanied by delayed bronchial complaints in 100%, especially by dyspnea and by delayed general complaints, especially pressure on the chest in 77% and tiredness in 100%.

(4) The DAR was associated with: delayed skin response in 63%, blood leucocytosis and slight lymphocytosis in 88%, but not blood eosinophilia, increased body temperature in 85%, and slight bradycardia in 71%.

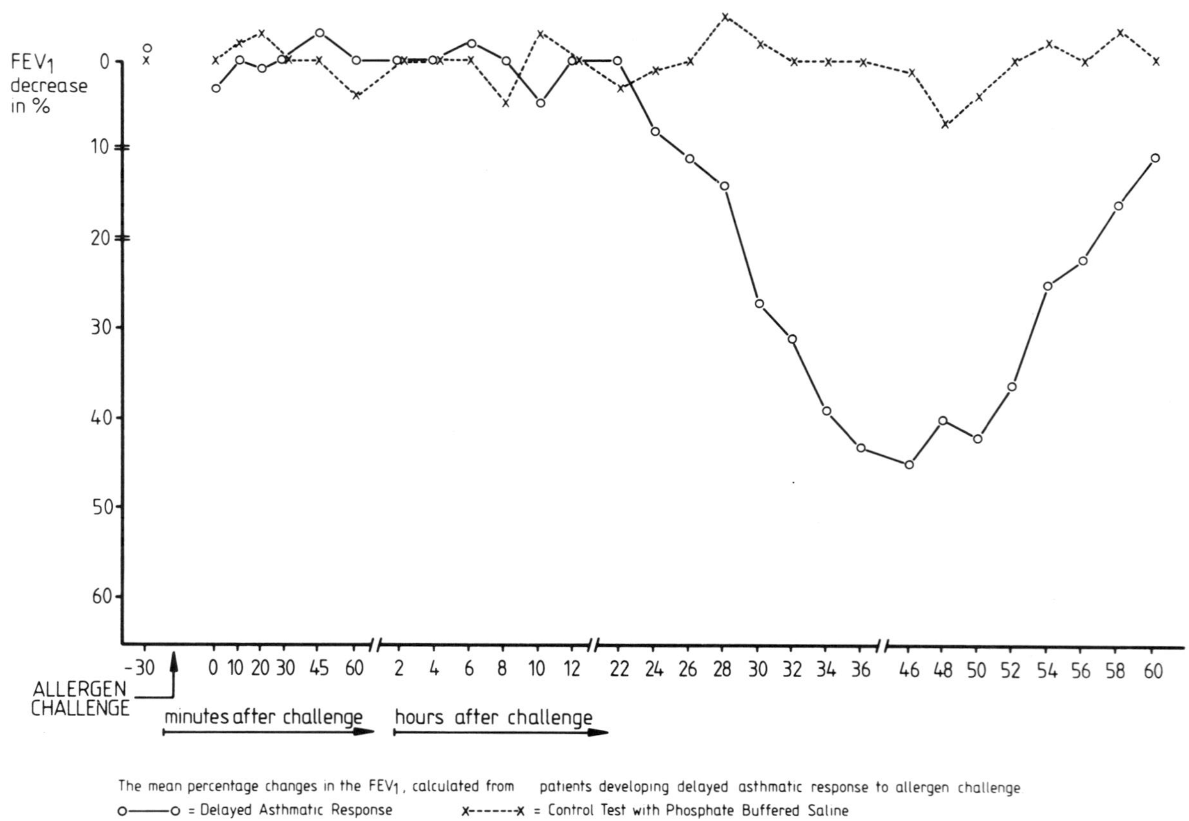

Fig. 1. Delayed asthmatic response (DAR) to allergen challenge.

The concentration of serum immunoglobulins was not significantly changed. No increased histamine concentration in the blood was detected in any of DAR cases.

(5) The responsiveness to histamine was increased only in 8% of the cases.

(6) The DAR was prevented distinctly by topical corticosteroids, Beclomethasone dipropionate and Budesonide, partially by Nedocromil Sodium, while Disodium cromoglycate and Salbutamol were ineffective (Table I).

Table I
Protective effects of the drugs on the DAR

DRUG	DAR n = 52
DISODIUM CROMOGLYCATE	-
NEDOCROMIL SODIUM	+
SALBUTAMOL	-
BECLOMETHASONE DIPROPIONATE	+++
BUDESONIDE	+++

Protective effects = - = no; ± = doubtful;
+ = slight; ++ = good; +++ = very good

CONCLUSION

An unusual, so-called "Delayed asthmatic response" (DAR), appearing between 24 and 56 (96) hours after allergen challenge, was recorded in 17% of the patients with allergic bronchial asthma. The association of DAR with other diagnostic parameters and accompanying clinical complaints as well as its pharmacologic control, were distinctly different from those observed in immediate (IAR) and late (LAR) asthmatic responses [1-3].

The exact mechanism(s) underlying the DAR is not yet known. With respect to the results of this study, however, the involvement of hypersensitivity mechanism(s) different from those presumed in the IAR and LAR, e.g. cell-mediated hypersensitivity, cannot be excluded.

REFERENCES

[1] Pelikan, Z., Pelikan-Filipek, M., Kruis, M., and Berger, M.P.F. (1986) The immediate asthmatic response to allergen challenge. Annals of Allergy, 56, 252-260.

[2] Pelikan, Z., Pelikan-Filipek, M. (1986) The late asthmatic response to allergen challenge, Part I + II. Annals of Allergy, 56, 414-420, 421-435.

[3] Pelikan, Z. (1989) Delayed asthmatic response and its pharmacological modulation. J. Allergy Clin. Immunol. 83, 244 (Abstr. 290).

[4] Siriganian, R.P. (1976) Histamine release and assay methods for the study of human allergy. In: Manual of Clinical Immunology, Rose, N.R., and Friedman, H., Eds., American Society for Microbiology, Washington (DC), 603-615.

CYTOLOGIC CHANGES IN THE NASAL SECRETIONS (NS) DURING THE IMMEDIATE (INR) AND LATE NASAL RESPONSE (LNR) TO ALLERGEN CHALLENGE (NPT)

Z. Pelikan and M. Pelikan-Filipek

Dept. of Allergology & Immunology, Inst. Med. Sci. "De Klokkenberg", Galderseweg 81, Breda, The Netherlands

INTRODUCTION

The purpose of this study was: (1) to investigate changes in the count of individual cell types in the nasal secretions and their relationship to the immediate and the late nasal response; (2) to determine the significance of the count of individual cell types and its changes for the INR and LNR; and criteria upon which those changes could be accepted as a supplementary diagnostic parameter.

The 221 patients with allergic rhinitis, developing 117 positive immediate (INR) and 104 late (LNR) nasal responses to challenge with "inhalant" allergens correlating with positive disease history and intradermal tests, and 60 patients demonstrating negative nasal responses (NNR) correlating with negative history and negative intradermal tests, were randomly selected for this study.

The nasal challenges were then repeated with the same allergens and supplemented by cytological examination of the nasal secretions. The cytological examination of NS was also performed during all control challenges with PBS (Phosphate Buffered Saline).

None of the patients studied has been treated by oral or topical corticosteroids, cromolyn or immunotherapy in the past, or by long acting antihistamines during the last 3 months.

Nasal provocation tests (NPT) were performed by means of rhinomanometry [1]. The parameters, the NPG values (nasopharynx-nostril-pressure gradients = Δ P), expressed in cm H_2O, were recorded before and up to 12 hours after the allergen challenge. The control challenge with PBS was performed in the same way as that with allergen [1].

Three series of the nasal secretions specimens were collected each time, by having the patient blow onto a polyethylene sheet twice before and 17 times after the allergen or PBS challenge.

The 1st series was stained by Hansel's method; the 2nd by modified May-Grünwald-Giemsa (MGG) method and the 3rd by Toluidine blue. The specimens were scanned microscopically by two counting techniques: (1) the differentiation count; (2) the counting of absolute numbers of the individual cell types per microscopic field (at magnification 25 x 12 = x 300), calculated always as a mean from 25 fields [2-4].

The results from MGG stained specimens were considered by us to be basic data.

Statistical analysis: (1) the nasal responses were evaluated by Wilcoxon matched paired signed rank test; (2) the changes in the count of particular cell types during the individual nasal responses by Wilcoxon paired test.

RESULTS

(1) The immediate nasal response (INR, n = 117) (Fig. 1):

(a) In most cases of INR the eosinophils, neutrophils, epithelial cells and goblet cells were found in the NS, while in some of them basophils and lymphocytes were also found. The mast cells, plasma cells and monocytes were recorded in NS during the INR only sporadically.

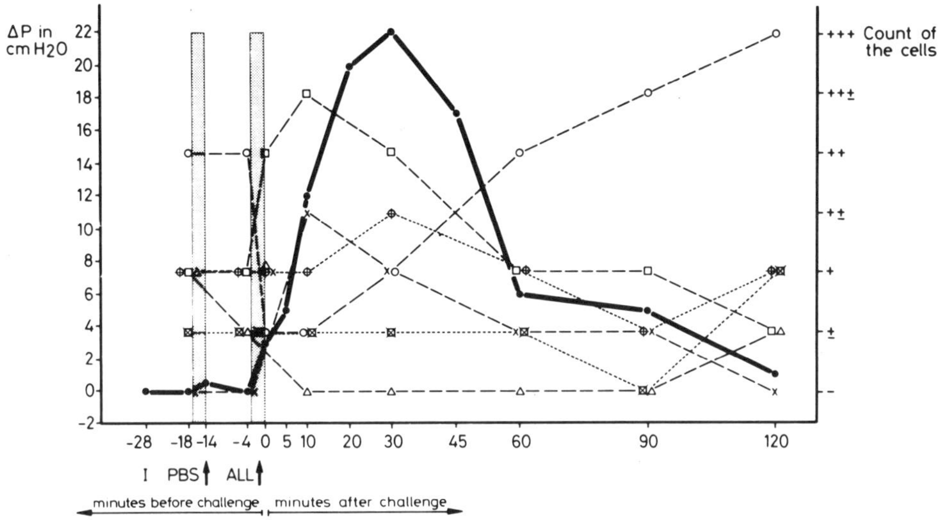

The mean NPG values, recorded after the allergen challenge with respect to the appropriate "PBS NPG values, were calculated from all 117 positive immediate nasal responses (+INR).
The mean changes in the count of the individual types of cells in the nasal secretions, were always calculated only from those INRs, during which the cells were present in the nasal secretions (see percentage-number in parasynthesis).

●▬▬● = +INR = positive immediate nasal response (n = 117 = 100 %)
□– – –□ = ES = eosinophils (in 85% of +INRs)
△– – –△ = BS = basophils (in 16% of +INRs)
○– – –○ = NT = neutrophils (in 91% of +INRs)
x– – –x = GC = goblet cells (in 87% of +INRs)
⊠········⊠ = LT = lymphocytes (in 11% of +INRs)
⊕········⊕ = EC = epithelial cells (in 68% of +INRs)
I = initial value PBS = PBS value ALL = allergen challenge

Fig. 1. The changes in the cell-counts in the nasal secretions during the positive immediate nasal response to allergen challenge (+INR).

(b) The INR was accompanied by significant changes in the count of eosinophils in 68% of the cases (increase followed by decrease), neutrophils in 43% (decrease followed by increase), goblet cells in 48% (increase followed by decrease) and basophils in 16% (decrease) in the NS. The other cell types (epithelial cells, monocytes, plasma cells and mast cells) did not demonstrate any significant changes in their count in the NS during the INR (Table I).

(2) The late nasal response (LNR, n = 104) (Fig. 2):

(a) In most cases of LNR, the epithelial cells, neutrophils, goblet cells and eosinophils were found in the NS, while in some of them basophils and lymphocytes were also found. The other cell types appeared in NS during the LNR irregularly.

Table I
Presence of individual cell types in the nasal secretions and changes in their count during the positive INR in %.

INR n = 117	Presence of the cells	Changes in the cell count before and after allergen
EOSINOPHILS	85	68*
NEUTROPHILS	91	43*
BASOPHILS	16	16
EPITHELIAL CELLS	68	11*
GOBLET CELLS	87	48*
LYMPHOCYTES	11	2
MAST CELLS	4	0
PLASMA CELLS	7	0
MONOCYTES	3	0

* statistically significant

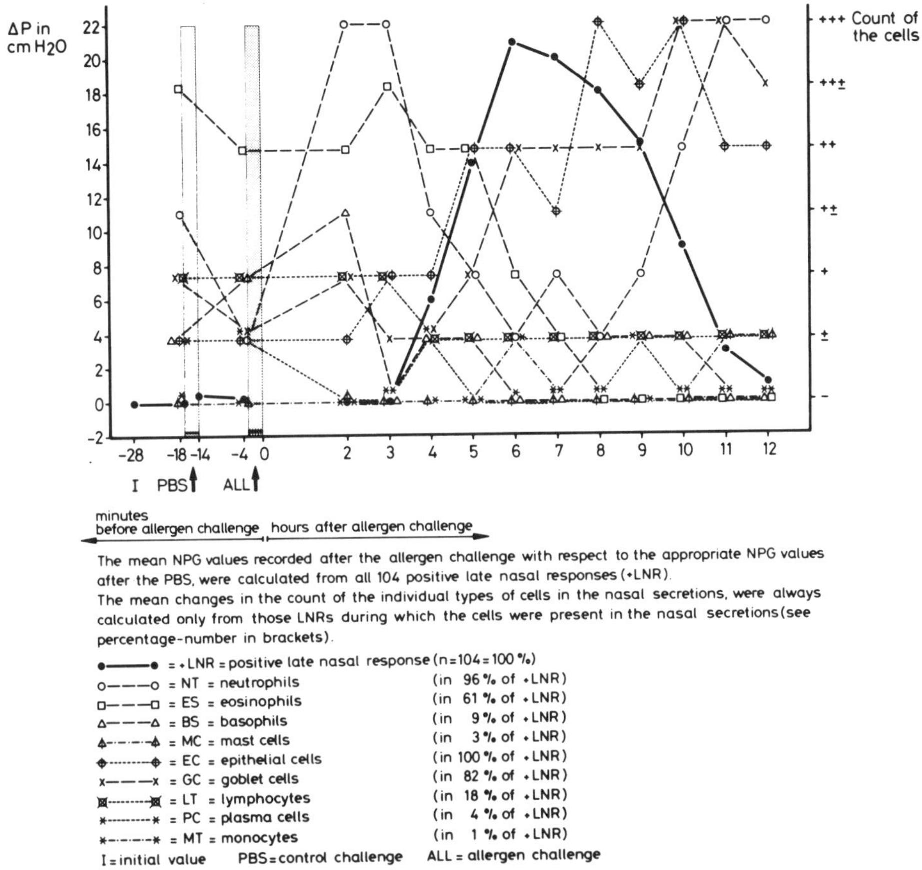

Fig. 2. The changes in the cell-counts in the nasal secretions during the positive late nasal response to allergen challenge (+LNR).

b) The LNR was accompanied by significant changes in the count of neutrophils in 84% of the cases (increase before, decrease during appearance and increase during resolving of the LNR), eosinophils in 58% (increase before and decrease during appearance of the LNR), epithelial cells in 73% (increase followed by decrease, running parallel with the clinical course of the LNR), goblet cells in 63% (increase followed by decrease) basophils in 8% (decrease) and lymphocytes in 6% (decrease) (Table II).

(3) <u>Negative nasal responses (NNR; n = 60) and PBS control challenges (PBS; n = 281)</u>: Were accompanied by presence of the individual cell types in the NS only in a minority of cases. No significant changes were recorded in the count of the particular cell types in the NS during the NNR nor during the PBS controls (Table III).

<u>Table II</u>
Presence of individual cell types in the nasal secretions and changes in their count during the positive LNR in %.

LNR n = 104	Presence of the cells	Changes in the cell count before and after allergen
EOSINOPHILS	61	58*
NEUTROPHILS	96	84*
BASOPHILS	15	8*
EPITHELIAL CELLS	100	73*
GOBLET CELLS	82	63*
LYMPHOCYTES	18	6*
MAST CELLS	3	0
PLASMA CELLS	4	0
MONOCYTES	1	0

* statistically significant

Table III
Presence of individual cell types in the nasal secretions and changes in their count during the negative response (NNR) in %.

NNR n = 60	Presence of the cells	Changes in the cell count before and after allergen
EOSINOPHILS	19	5
NEUTROPHILS	17	3
BASOPHILS	9	0
EPITHELIAL CELLS	23	7
GOBLET CELLS	13	4
LYMPHOCYTES	4	3
MAST CELLS	2	0
PLASMA CELLS	2	0
MONOCYTES	0	0

CONCLUSIONS

(I) A single recording of the cells in nasal secretions (NS) is not a suitable diagnostic parameter. The cells in NS should be recorded before and repeatedly after the nasal challenge with a certain allergen and only the changes in their count should be considered as a supplementary diagnostic parameter [1-4].

(II) The positive INR and LNR were associated with changes in the count of individual cell types in NS to different degrees and patterns. These results may suggest: firstly: different involvement and role of the individual cell types in both types of nasal responses; and secondly: the possibility of involvement of different hypersensitivity mechanisms in the INR and LNR [1-5].

REFERENCES

[1] Pelikan, Z. (1978) Late and delayed responses of the nasal mucosa to allergen challenge. Annals of Allergy, 41, 37-47.

[2] Pelikan, Z. (1983) The changes in the nasal secretions of eosinophils during the immediate nasal response to allergen challenge. J. Allergy Clin. Immunol., 83, 1068-1079.

[3] Pelikan, Z., and Pelikan-Filipek, M. (1988) Cytologic changes in the nasal secretions during the immediate nasal response. J. Allergy Clin. Immunol., 82, 1103-1112.

[4] Pelikan Z., and Pelikan-Filipek M. (1989) Cytologic changes in the nasal secretions during the late nasal response. J. Allergy Clin. Immunol., 83, 1068-1079.

[5] Pelikan Z. (1979) The role of immediate, late, and delayed reactions in allergic nasal disease. In: J. Pepys and A.M. Edwards, eds, The mast cell, its role in health and disease. Proceedings of an International Symposium, Davos, April, 23-26, 1979 (Switzerland), Pitman Medical, Tunbridge Wells (UK), 772-777.

AAS 31:
Mediators in
Airway Hyperreactivity

AIRWAY DIAMETER DETERMINES FLOW-RESISTANCE AND SENSITIVITY TO CONTRACTILE MEDIATORS IN PERFUSED BRONCHIAL SEGMENTS

M.P. Sparrow, K.E. Willet and H.W. Mitchell

Department of Physiology, University of Western Australia, Nedlands 6009, Australia

SUMMARY: To study airway reactivity, flow-resistance to carbachol and histamine was measured in perfused bronchial segments. Small-bore airways were more sensitive, flow was reduced to zero and resistance rose very steeply due to mucosal folding while in large-bore airways maximum flow reduction was 50% and resistance increased sigmoidly. Thus the internal diameter of an airway is a crucial determinant of narrowing.

Bronchial hyperreactivity (BH) is seen as excessive narrowing of the airways in response to stimuli. The magnitude of narrowing in vitro can be measured using the perfused bronchial segment (Mitchell et al.,1989; Mitchell and Sparrow,1990) shown in Fig. 1. In contrast to isolated strips of bronchial wall the perfused bronchial segment retains the essential features which determine the extent of narrowing, namely, the diameter of the lumen, the wall geometry, the epithelium forming a continuous lining around the lumen and the transmural pressure. We describe here the effect of the airway diameter (and how it influences the wall geometry) on the responses to mediators.

RESULTS AND DISCUSSION

When a small-bore segment of internal diameter (i.d.) 2.5mm was perfused (Fig. 1), it narrowed rapidly in response to electrical stimulation of the intramural nerves as shown by a reduction in

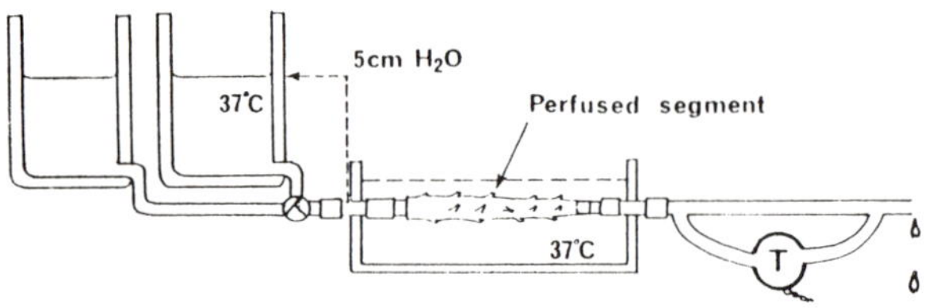

Fig. 1. A 3.5 cm segment from the stem bronchus (between branches #15-20) of the lung of a pig (26 weeks) was cannulated and perfused with Krebs at a constant pressure head of $5cmH_2O$ (see Mitchell et al.,1989) and the flow rate measured with a Motorola MDX10DP transducer. Contractile mediators were introduced into the perfusate or into the organ bath. Intramural nerves were stimulated using platinum ring electrodes. When the perfused segment was relaxed using theophylline 10mM or fully contracted with carbachol (still at $5cmH_2O$) it was instantly frozen in isopentane precooled in liquid N_2 and sections were cut for morphometry and muscle shortening (James et al.,1988).

Fig. 2

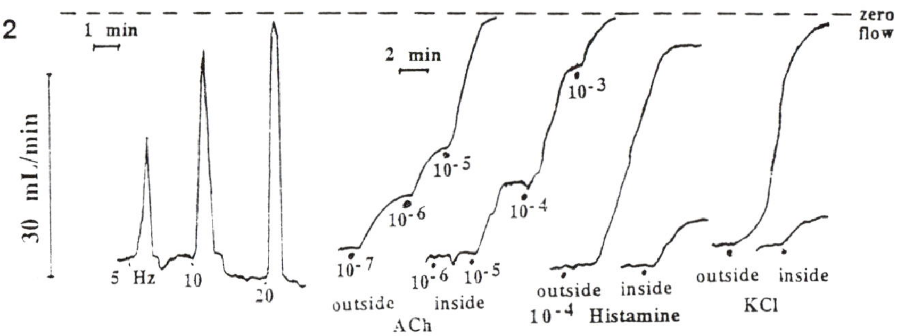

flow rate (Fig. 2). At 20 Hz, 0.5msec the flow almost ceased, i.e. the lumen had virtually closed off. The sensitivity of acetylcholine, histamine and KCl (replacing the NaCl in Krebs) was much greater when applied on the outside than via the lumen. Fig. 3 compares concentration-flow curves to carbachol and histamine perfused through the lumen. Carbachol displayed the greater sensitivity (EC_{50} 8.5μM vs 63μM) but both reduced flow to zero. By plotting as resistance (Fig. 3b) (pressure/flow) the extent of narrowing was more strikingly demonstrated where a rise in resistance occurred which was approximately exponential.

Fig. 3

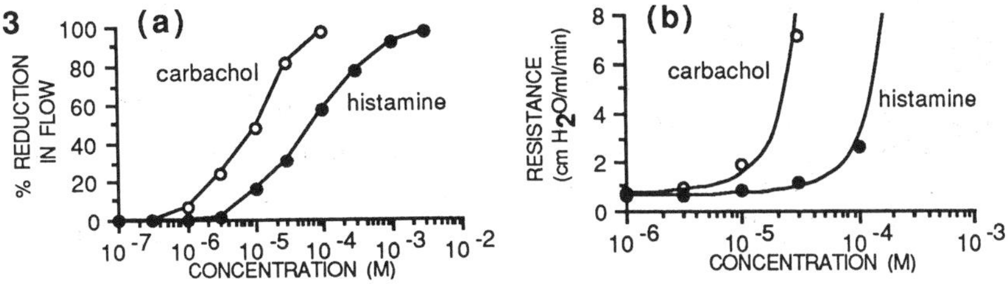

Figure 4a compares small and large-bore airways. Bronchial segments of 2.6mm i.d.(at the distal end) narrowed to the point where flow ceased but in 5.4mm i.d. segments flow was reduced by 50% at a maximum concentration of carbachol (and also with histamine, not shown). The resistance changes contrasted sharply (Fig. 4b) with the concentration-resistance curves being approximately exponential in the small airway and sigmoidal in the

Fig. 4

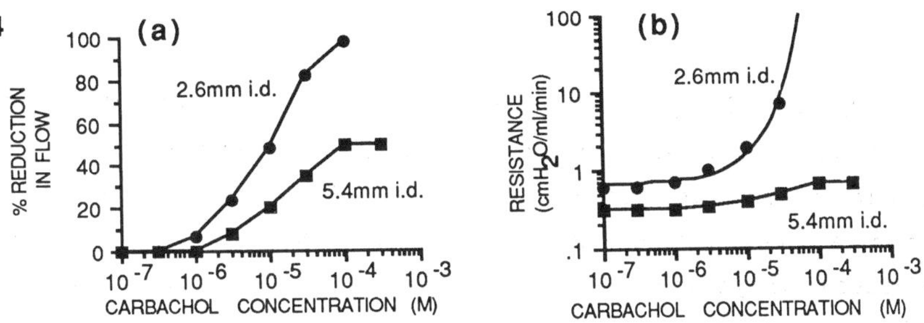

large airway. The smooth muscle shortened by 27% of its initial resting length in the small-bore airway causing the lumen to be almost entirely obstructed by the extensively folded mucosa. In contrast in the large-bore airway where the resistance changes were quite small the muscle shortened by 37%, significantly greater than in the small airway ($P< 0.05$) and the extent of mucosal folding was quite small.

The concentration-flow or resistance curves reported here in response to spasmogens are highly dependant on the internal diameter of the airway. Furthermore they bear little resemblance to the concentration-response curves obtained from strips of

Fig. 5

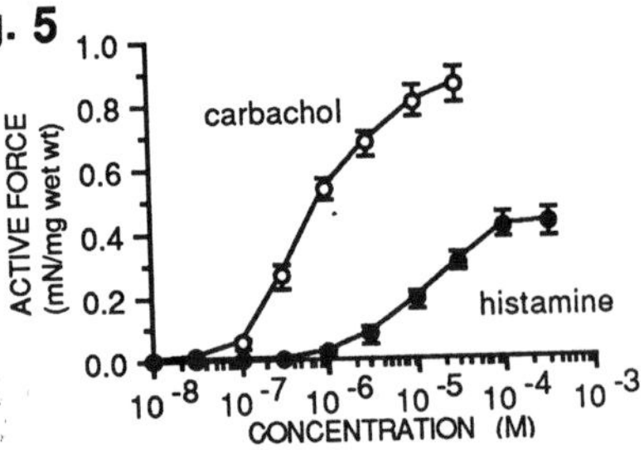

bronchial wall which are so frequently used to characterise the effects of mediators. Fig. 5 shows that bronchial strips from the same pig lungs are more sensitive to carbachol than histamine (EC_{50} = 0.60μM vs 11.5μM) and the Emax is doubled. But the Emax has no counterpart in the small-bore bronchial segment preparation where both agents reduce flow to zero. Furthermore histamine 10^{-4}M to 10^{-3}M is maximum in strips but on the inside of the tubular segment closes it off (Fig. 3). This shows that at forces above 0.4mN/mg wet weight in strips the airway is fully narrowed so that the upper part of the concentration-response curve to carbachol is not necessarily relevant to airway narrowing.

CONCLUSION: The perfused bronchial segment provides a means of investigating the effects of mediators on airway narrowing using an isolated section of the bronchial tree. The internal diameter of the airway (and inter alia the mucosal folding and wall thickness) plays a crucial role in determining the characteristics of flow-resistance.

REFERENCES

Mitchell, H.W., Willet K.W. and Sparrow M.P. (1989), Perfused segment and bronchial strip: narrowing vs isometric force by mediators. J. Appl.Physiol. 66, 2704-2709.

Mitchell, H.W. and Sparrow, M.P. (1989), The relevance of pharmacological dose-response curves to airway narrowing. Trends in Pharmacological Sciences. 10, 488-491.

James, A.L., Hogg, J.C., Dunn, L.A. and Pare, P.D. (1988), The use of the internal perimeter to compare airway size and to calculate smooth muscle shortening. Am. Rev. Resp. Dis. 138, 136-139.

AAS 31:
Mediators in
Airway Hyperreactivity

MODULATING EFFECTS OF ANTIASTHMATIC AND ANTITUSSIVE DRUGS ON AUTONOMIC NEUROTRANSMISSION IN GUINEA-PIG BRONCHIAL MUSCLE IN VITRO.

Y. Kamikawa and Y. Shimo.

Department of Pharmacology, Dokkyo University School of Medicine
Mibu, Tochigi 321-02, Japan.

SUMMARY: Electrical field stimulation evoked a biphasic contraction of the guinea-pig isolated bronchi, consisting of a cholinergically mediated fast contraction followed by a non-cholinergically mediated slow contraction. Catecholamines, β_2-stimulants, methylxanthines, antiallergic drugs, narcotic and non-narcotic antitussive drugs inhibited the neurogenic contractions not only by postjunctional depression of the response but also by prejunctional reduction of the transmitter release.

INTRODUCTION

Recent evidence indicates that guinea-pig peripheral airways are predominantly innervated by excitatory cholinergic and non-cholinergic nerves and that substance P (SP) or neurokinin A (NKA) might function as the transmitter substance of the non-cholinergic nerves (Andersson & Grundstrom, 1987). The tachykinin-containing nerves are thought to be sensory nerves in origin and to have a potential role for producing cough and bronchoconstriction as a defens reflex. The aim of the present study was to investigate the modulating effects of antiasthmatic and antitussive drugs on electrically induced neurogenic contractions of the guinea-pig bronchi.

MATERIALS AND METHODS

Preparation: Male guinea-pigs (300-700 g) were stunned, the tracheo-bronchial tree excised and the bronchial strip chain was prepared (Kamikawa & Shimo, 1989). The strip was immersed in a 10 ml organ bath filled with modified Krebs bicarbonate solution containing 20 μM choline chloride and 2 μM indomethacin (pH 7.4), and was bubled with a 5% CO_2 - 95% O_2 mixture at 37°C. The preparation was suspended under an initial tension of 0.5 g and the bronchial response was isometrically recorded by means of a force-displacement transducer and a polygraph recorder (Nihon Kohden, SB-1T-H and RJG-4004).

Electrical field stimulation: Electrical field stimulation was with rectangular pulses of 8Hz frequency, 0.5 msec duration, 40 pulses and supramaximal voltage, through bipolar platinum electrodes connected to a Nihon Kohden stimulator (SEN-1011). When the strip was electrically stimulated, a biphasic contraction was obtained, composed of an initial fast contraction mediated by cholinergic- followed by a sustained contraction mediated by non-cholinergic-nerve stimulation. The height of these contraction were comparable to those of submaximal contractions induced by exogenous acetylcholine (ACh, 2 μM) and SP (0.2 μM) or NKA (10 nM), respectively.

RESULTS

Catecholamines: Both adrenaline and isoproterenol inhibited the electrically induced neurogenic contractions where non-cholinergic component was more potently inhibited than cholinergic component. Although the inhibitory action of isoproterenol was mostly reversed by propranolol alone, that of adrenaline was only partly reversed by propranolol alone, but was mostly reversed by the further addition of yohimbine (Kamikawa & Shimo, 1990).

β_2-Stimulants: Salbutamol, terbutaline, clenbuterol, fenoterol and procaterol inhibited the electrically induced non-cholinergic contraction more than cholinergic contraction, where procaterol was the most potent. These β_2-stimulants inhibited the ACh-induced contraction more than the SP-induced contraction. These inhibitory actions were reversed by propranolol alone.

Methylxanthines: Aminophylline and enprofylline fairly inhibited the electrically induced neurogenic contractions and the ACh- or SP-induced contractions.

Anticholinergic drug: Ipratropium bromide selectively inhibited the electrically induced cholinergic contraction and the ACh-induced contraction.

Antiallergic drugs: Sodium cromoplycate showed a weak but selective inhibition of the non-cholinergic contraction. Among orally active antiallergic drugs, tranilast and azelastine inhibited the non-cholinergic contraction more than cholinergic contraction, while ketotifen more potently inhibited the cholinergic contraction (Kamikawa, 1989).

Narcotic antitussive drugs: Morphine and BW443C selectively inhibited the non-cholinergic contraction, without any inhibition on the ACh- or SP-induced contraction. The inhibitory actions were mostly reversed by naloxone (Kamikawa & Shimo, 1990).

Non-narcotic antitussive drugs: Ephedrine, dextromethorphan, noscapine and tipepidine fairly inhibited both cholinergic and non-cholinergic contractions where tipepidine was the most potent. Submaximal contractions to SP or NKA were unaffected by these drugs.

DISCUSSION

In this study we have demonstrated that all antiasthmatic and antitussive drugs tested inhibited the electrically induced neurogenic contractions of guinea-pig bronchial muscle. The inhibitory potencies, however, were variable not only among the drugs but also between cholinergic and non-cholinergic component of the response. Catecholamines, β_2-stimulants, antiallergic drugs and opioids more strongly inhibited the non-cholinergic contraction than the cholinergic contraction, whereas ipratropium, ketotifen and tipepidine more strongly inhibited the cholinergic contraction. Since these drugs inhibited submaximal contractions to exogenous ACh, SP or NKA less than those to electrical stimulation, their inhibitory effects on neurogenic contractions are thought to be preferentially mediated by prejunctional reduction of the transmitter release and partly by postjunctional depression on bronchial muscle. The present results indicate that non-cholinergic neurotransmission may be an important target for antiasthmatic and antitussive drugs.

REFERENCES

Andersson, R.G.G. and Grundstrom, N. (1987) Innervation of airway smooth muscle. Pharmacol. Therap. 32, 107-130.

Kamikawa, Y. and Shimo, Y. (1989) Adenosine selectively inhibits non-cholinergic transmission in guinea pig bronchi. J. Appl. Physiol. 66, 2084-2091.

Kamikawa, Y. (1989) Inhibitory effect of anti-allergic drugs on cholinergic and non-cholinergic neurotransmissions of guinea pig bronchial muscle in vitro. Ann. Allergy 63, 59-63.

Kamikawa, Y. and Shimo, Y. (1990) Inhibitory effects of catecholamines on cholinergically and non-cholinergically mediated contractions of guinea-pig isolated bronchial muscle. J.Pharm. Pharmacol. 42, 131-134.

Kamikawa, Y. and Shimo, Y. (1990) Morphine and opioid peptides selectively inhibit the non-cholinergic contraction of guinea-pig bronchial muscle, J. Pharm. Pharmacol. 42, 214-216.

EFFECT OF SUBACUTE EXPOSURE TO NITROGEN DIOXIDE ON THE AIRWAY RESPONSIVENESS OF GUINEA PIG

TAKAHIRO KOBAYASHI and YUMI SHINOZAKI

Department of Basic Medical Sciences, The National Institute for Environmental Studies and Medical Sciences, University of Tsukuba, Tsukuba, Ibaraki 305, Japan.

SUMMARY: Subacute (7 days) exposure of guinea pigs to 4 ppm NO_2 induces transient airway hyperresponsiveness to inhaled histamine (His)-aerosol as does acute exposure to higher concentration of NO_2. Thromboxane A_2 may play an important role in this transient airway hyperresponsiveness.

Nitrogen dioxide (NO_2) is a major component of air pollution in urban areas. The effect of subacute and chronic exposure to NO_2 on airway responsiveness has remained to be elucidated. The mechanism of airway hyperresponsiveness induced by exposure to NO_2 has also remained to be elucidated. Therefore, in order to clarify the relationship between exposure to NO_2 and asthma, we investigated, 1) whether subacute exposure of guinea pigs to 4 ppm NO_2 could increase their airway responsiveness to inhaled His-aerosol and, if so, 2) whether thromboxane A_2 may be involved in the airway hyperresponsiveness induced by subacute exposure to this gas.

MATERIALS AND METHODS

Protocol: Female Hartley guinea pigs were used. On day 0, baseline specific airway resistance (SRaw) and airway responsiveness to inhaled His-aerosol were measured. On day 7, the animals were exposed to NO_2 or filtered air (Kobayashi et al., 1983) after having been divided into 6 groups (n=15 each). Three groups were exposed to filtered air for 1, 3, or 7 days (24 h/day); and the other three groups to 4 ppm NO_2 for 1, 3, or 7 days (24 h/day). On the day of termination of exposure, airway responsiveness to inhaled His-aerosol was determined.

Measurement of SRaw: SRaw was measured in a constant-volume body plethysmograph based on the design of Agrawal (1981).

Airway responsiveness: Airway responsiveness was assessed by measurement of SRaw as a function of increasing concentration of His. Saline and His-aerosol were generated by nebulizers (NE-U11B, Omron, Tokyo) containing 0.0, 0.1, 0.25, 0.5, 1.0, 2.5, 5.0, and 10.0 mM His in saline. The effective Molar concentration of His (EC_{200} His) that produced a doubling of $SRaw_{NaCl}$ (SRaw after inhalation of 0.9% NaCl aerosol) was determined by interpolation.

RESULTS

Effect of NO_2 exposure on baseline specific airway resistance, $SRaw_0$: Comparison of $SRaw_0$ determined 1 week before inhalation with that measured immediately after inhalation of 4 ppm NO_2 or filtered air for 1, 3, or 7 days revealed that $SRaw_0$ did not change significantly.

Effects of NO_2 exposure on airway responsiveness: Prior to exposure to NO_2 for 1, 3, or 7 days, EC_{200}His, concentrations of inhaled His necessary to double $SRaw_{NaCl}$ were 1.07 ± 0.20, 1.30 ± 0.20, and 1.01 ± 0.18 mM respectively. The corresponding values post-exposure were 1.42 ± 0.25, 0.66 ± 0.10, and 1.05 ± 0.22 mM. The results show that a 3 day exposure to NO_2 caused a significant increase in airway responsiveness to inhaled His-aerosol ($P<0.05$). Exposure to filtered air alone had no significant effect on the airway responsiveness to inhaled His-aerosol.

Comparison of airway responsiveness in pre- and post-exposure to NO_2 or air: Comparison of EC_{200}His values between pre- and post-exposure to NO_2 or air were compared in each animal. Animals showing a decrease or an increase in EC_{200}His to under half or above twice that of the pre-exposure values were considered hyperresponsive or hyporesponsive, respectively. After exposure to NO_2 for 1, 3, or 7 days, 4, 11, and 2 of the 15 animals in each group became hyperresponsive, and 4, 1 and 2 became hyporesponsive, respectively. In the groups exposed to filtered air for 1, 3 or 7 days, 2, 1, and 1 of the 15 guinea pigs of each group became hyperresponsive, and 2, 3, and 2 became hyporesponsive, respectively.

Effect of OYY 046 on NO_2-induced airway hyperresponsiveness: OKY 046 had no significant effect on airway responsiveness to inhaled His-aerosol after exposure to filtered air. In the animals exposed for 3 days to 4 ppm NO_2 and then subjected to OKY 046 inhalation, airway responsiveness to inhaled His-aerosol also did not change significantly (1.37 ± 0.31 mM pre vs. 1.24 ± 0.30 mM post). Thus, thromboxane A_2 would appear to play an important role in the development of airway hyper-responsiveness following NO_2 exposure.

DISCUSSION

The results of this study showed that even lower concentrations of NO_2 than those previously reported (Silbaugh et al., 1981) can induce transient hyperresponsiveness in experimental animals after an appropriate long-term exposure. A previous report based on a study in dogs showed that thromboxane A_2 may be an important mediator of O_3-induced airway hyperresponsiveness (Aizawa et al., 1985). As OKY 046 inhibited the induction of airway hyperresponsiveness by 3-days exposure to NO_2 in our study, thromboxane A_2 would appear to be an important mediator of NO_2-induced airway hyperresponsiveness. NO_2 induced airway hyperresponsiveness, which responsiveness then decreased and returned to the normal level even when the NO_2 exposure continued. A mechanism to explain the decrease in the increased airway responsiveness can be postulated. Increased secretion by airway cells may have caused the decrease in the penetration of the inhaled histamine have caused the decrease in the increased airway hyperresponsiveness. The tendency toward an increase in $SRaw_0$ after exposure to 4 ppm NO_2 for 7 days may support this possibility.

Our results also show that 1) the time course of change in airway response differs individually, and 2) facility of the induction or airway hyperresponsiveness also differs individually. Therefore the population in whom airway hyperresponsiveness is easily induced by an air pollutant such as NO_2 appear to be the high risk population in the outbreak of asthmatic symptoms elicited by air pollutants.

ACKNOWLEDGMENTS: OKY 046 was generously donated by Ono Pharmaceuticals Co. Ltd. (Osaka, Japan). Supported in part by Grant-in-Aid (No.62570354) C for Scientific Research from the Ministry of Education, Science and Culture of Japan.

REFERENCES:

Agrawal, K.P. (1981) Special airway conductance in guinea pigs: Normal values and histamine induced fall. Respir. Physiol. 43, 23-30.

Aizawa, H, Chung, K.F., Leikauf, G.D., Ueki, I., Bethel, R.A., O'Byrne, P.M., Hirose, T., and Nadel, J.A. (1985) Significance of thromboxane generation in ozone-induced airway hyperresponsiveness in dogs. J. Appl. Physiol. 59, 1918-1923.

Kobayashi, T., Morita, I., and Murota, S. (1983) Effects of nitrogen dioxide exposure on prostacyclin synthesis in lung and thromboxane A_2 synthesis in platelets in rats. Prostaglandins 26, 303-310.

Silbaugh, S.A., Mauderly, J.L., Macken, C.A. (1981) Effects of sulfuric acid and nitrogen dioxide on airway responsiveness of the guinea pig. J. Toxicol. Environm. Health 8, 31-45.

TOXOCARA CANIS-INDUCED AIRWAY HYPOREACTIVITY IN MICE

J. Buijs *, M.W.E.C.Egbers** and F.P.Nijkamp**

* Inst.of Public Health and Environmental Hygiene,Lab.Parasitology and Mycology, P.O.Box 1, 3720 BA, Bilthoven, The Netherlands

**Fac.of Pharmacy, Dept.of Pharmacology, Utrecht University, Catharijnesingel 60, 3511 GH, Utrecht

SUMMARY: Migrating larvae of the canine nematode Toxocara canis induce inflammatory responses in the lungs of infected mice. Histological examination of the lungs showed that mice developed persistent multifocal inflammation in which eosinophils (eos), macrophages (Mϕ) and many lymphocytes were involved. Cuffing of bloodvessels and bronchioles with mixed cell populations was also observed. Investigation into the response of isolated tracheae to cholinergic and β-adrenergic receptor agonists demonstrated a significant decreased reactivity despite the pronounced involvement of eos and Mϕ. This hyporeactive state persisted for ≥4 weeks p.i..

INTRODUCTION: The 2nd stage larvae of the canine nematode Toxocara canis are the cause of visceral larva migrans (VLM) in man and animals. In canines only the infective stage grows sexually mature. In the non-specific host they remain in the phase of tissue migrating larvae. Infection in man may cause disease, the VLM syndrome (VLMS) . Symptoms are a.o. fever, wheezing, pneumonitis, eosinophilia (Glickman and Schantz, 1981), and polyclonal activation of IgE producing B cells (Nutman et al,1984). A relation between parasitic infections and the occurrence of bronchial asthma was suggested (Woodruff,1970). Experiments with the Toxocara related ascarid Ascaris suum showed that a hyperreactive state may develop during infection (Johnson and Stout, 1989;). The aim of the presented study was to investigate whether or not a primary Toxocara infection in mice affects airway smooth muscle. Parallel to airway smooth muscle reactivity the histo-pathology of the lungs was studied. Mice were chosen as experimental animals as mouse VLM has much in common with human VLM (Kayes 1984).

MATERIALS AND METHODS

Experimental animals: Male BALB/c mice (spf), 6-8 weeks old, RIVM, Bilthoven, The Netherlands.
Toxocara canis: The T.canis strain has been maintained in dogs since 1986. Eggs collected from the uteri of adult female worms were processed as described by Kayes (1984). Mice were infected with 1000 infective eggs/animal. Infection was given by oral intubation.
Histology: The animals were sacrificed using Nembutal (60 mg/kg i.p.) as anaestheticum. The abdomen and chest were opened. The lungs were perfused with saline and removed.They were intratracheally inoculated with 4% formalin and immersed in the same fixative. The tissue was processed using a Tissue Tek vacuum infiltration processor,(Bayer/Miles). 5μm Sections were stained according to convential methods i.e. Haemaluin Eosine (HE), Giemsa-May Grünwald (MG) and Periodic Acid Schiff (PAS).
Trachea isolation and measurement: After anaesthesia (Nembutal 60mg/kg) the tracheae were removed and dissected free of irrelevant tissue. Carbachol and isoprenaline dose-response curves on mouse trachea were performed as described by Garssen et al (1990).

RESULTS

Histology: The lungs of the mice showed a multifocal inflammatory response. At 3 days p.i. the larvae had passed the lungs inducing haemorrhage and inflammation with mainly polymorphonuclears (PMN). The initially exsudative reaction was characterized by multifocal inflammatory sites populated with many eos, lymphocytes and Mϕ (Fig.1).
The bronchial epithelial cells of bronchiae and bronchioles were PAS positive suggesting increased mucus production. Perivascular and partial peribronchial cuffing with mixed cell populations was observed . From day 14 p.i. many plasmacells were present. The inflammation persisted until the end of the observation period which was at 90 days p.i.
Trachea smooth muscle cell reactivity: The carbachol dose-response curves demonstrated a significant decreased response of the trachea smooth muscle cells at days 7,14 and 28 p.i. At day 3 p.i. the reactivity did not differ from that of the non-infected animals (Fig.2).Also the response to isoprenaline was significantly decreased at days 7, 14 and 28 p.i..

DISCUSSION

The histological and pharmacological changes which were demonstrated to occur during a Toxocara canis infection seem paradoxical. The histological data presented would fit the criteria defined for bronchial asthma whereas the observed decrease in trachea reactivity contrast it. In addition to the presented results also total serum IgE increased significantly (results not shown). Different mechanisms may explain the observations. Inflammatory cells are present in large numbers. Toxic O_2metabolites produced by these cells may have caused damage to

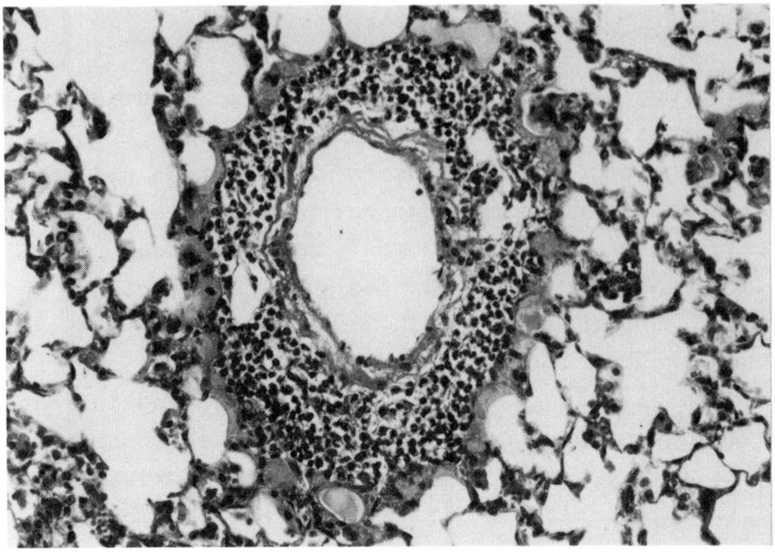

Fig. 1: Cross section through mouse lung 7 days post infection with 1000 Toxocara canis eggs. Small venule with several circular layers of a mixed cell population (= cuffing).

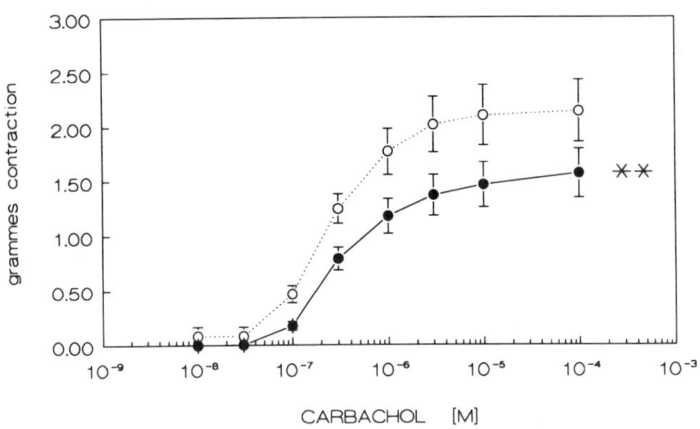

Fig. 2 Mean carbachol dose-response curve of isolated mouse trachea performed 14 days post infection with 1000 Toxocara canis eggs. The mean trachea reactivity of the infected group (—•—) is significant ($p < 0.01$) lower than that of the non-infected (--o--) group (the mean EC 50 values did not differ).

receptors with as a consequence unresponsiveness to their agonists. Another possibility is that the multifocal inflammation as such induced a decrease in the contraction/relaxation potential. Pleading against this suggestion is that infected guinea pigs were also hyporeactive to histamine although they showed only focal inflammation. Johnson and Stout (1989) found, using the model Ascaris suum in monkeys, that a hyperreactive response developed only after a challenge with specific antigen but not after histamine challenge. They argued that repeated contact with the specific antigen is needed for the development of a hyperreactive state. This may indicate that a primary Toxocara infection is an addition to the risk factors already known to induce non-specific bronchial asthma.

CONCLUSION

A primary Toxocara canis infection in mice induces an inflammatory reaction in the lungs. Despite the participation of eosinophils, macrophages and lymphocytes the trachea smooth muscle responded hyporeactive to both cholinergic and β-adrenergic receptor agonists.

REFERENCES

Garssen, J., Loveren, H.van, Vliet, H,van der and Nijkamp, F.P. (1990) An isometric method to study respiratory smooth muscle response in mice. J. Pharm. Meth. (in press)

Glickman, L.T., Schantz, P.M. (1981), Epidemiology and pathogenesis of zoonotic toxocariasis. Epidemiol. Rev. 3, 230-250

Johnson, H.G., and Stout, B.K. (1989), Ascaris suum ova-induced bronchoconstriction, eosinophilia and IgE antibody responses in experimentally infected primates did not lead to histamine hyperreactivity. Am. Rev. Resp. Dis. 139, 710-714

Kayes, S.G. (1984), Spleen cell responses in experimental murine toxocariasis. J. Parasit. 70, 522-529

Nutman, T.B., Hussain, R, and Ottesen, E.A. (1984), IgE production in vitro by peripheral blood mononuclear

cells of patients with parasitic helminth infections. Clin. Exp. Immunol. 58, 174-182
Woodruff, A.W. (1970), Toxocariasis. Br. Med. J. 19 Sept. 663-669

PLASTICISERS, ANOTHER BURDEN FOR ASTHMATICS ?

Cees J.A. Doelman, Paul J.A. Borm* and Aalt Bast.

Department of Pharmacochemistry, Faculty of Chemistry, Vrije Universiteit, De Boelelaan 1083, 1081 HV Amsterdam, The Netherlands.

* Department of Occupational & Environmental Health & Toxicology, State University of Limburg, P.O. Box 616, 6200 MD Maastricht, The Netherlands.

SUMMARY: The widely used plasticiser di(2-ethylhexyl)phthalate (DEHP) has been reported to have some toxicological effects on pulmonary tissue. Inhalation of DEHP may cause pulmonary edema and bronchial asthma. Moreover intravenous injection of DEHP induces pulmonary inflammation and hemorrhage of the lungs. We now report that DEHP might cause bronchial hyperresponsiveness. The metabolite of DEHP mono(2-ethylhexyl)phthalate (MEHP) induces in vitro a dose-dependent increase in -log EC_{50} for methacholine dose response curves in rat tracheal tissue. Moreover MEHP induces a decrease in maximal effect of the methacholine dose response curve. We concluded that DEHP due to the formation of MEHP in vivo, may cause bronchial hyperresponsiveness.

The flexibility of polyvinylchloride (PVC) plastics depends on the content of plasticiser. The mostly used plasticiser is di(2-ethylhexyl)phthalate (DEHP). PVC plastics may contain up to 40% of DEHP. Due to the extensive use of DEHP, it became a widespread environmental contaminant, present in food, soil, plants and bacteria. DEHP can even be detected in the atmosphere and therefore nobody escapes exposure. Workers in DEHP manufacture and patients recieving multiple blood transfusions are exposed to relatively high concentrations of DEHP. Blood plasma for intravenous injection may contain concentrations of DEHP up to 8 mg/100 ml when stored for longer periods (> 21 days) in medical disposable devices made from PVC plastics (Thomas et al., 1978).An increased risk of progressive respiratory failure has been associated with the use of stored bank blood (Bennett et al., 1972).

After intravenous administration, DEHP and its hydrolysis product mono(2-ethylhexyl)phthalate (MEHP) accumulate in the lungs. In rats, intravenous injection of DEHP results in pulmonary hemorrhage and inflammation followed by a sudden death (Schulz et al., 1975). DEHP has no effects after oral intake but inhalation of DEHP (for instance by the use of PVC-containing tracheal intubation systems) has been related to observed induction of pulmonary edema and bronchial asthma (Roth et al., 1988).

Because the mechanism of induction of bronchial asthma by DEHP is unclear, we tested the pharmacological effects of DEHP and its metabolites MEHP and phthalic acid on rat muscarinic receptor responses.

MATERIALS AND METHODS

Male Wistar rats (200-250 g, Harlan CPB, Zeist, The Netherlands) were used in this study. Rat tracheal strips were prepared according to the method described by Doelman et al.(1988). Muscarinic receptor responses were isotonically measured by the addition of cumulative doses of methacholine to the organ bath which contained a Krebs buffer solution (Doelman et al., 1988). After three dose response curves, tracheal strips were incubated for 30 min with DEHP, MEHP or phthalic acid, dissolved in 50 ml dimethylsulphoxide (DMSO) or incubated with 1(5-isoquinolinylsulphonyl)2-methylpiperazine (H7), dissolved in 50 ml ethanol. Methacholine dose response curves were measured in the presence of DEHP, MEHP, phthalic acid or H7. After a 60 min. washing period with 12 intermediate changes of buffer solution, again a methacholine dose response curve was recorded.

RESULTS

Methacholine dose response curves of rat tracheal tissue were not influenced by DEHP or phthalic acid (up to concentrations of 1mM) compared to the control (incubation with the solvent DMSO). As shown in figure 1 incubation with 10^{-4} M MEHP induced a significant increase in -log EC_{50} ($\pm$ s.e.m.) for methacholine compared to the control (5.63 ± 0.10 vs. 5.38 ± 0.04 respectively). No change in maximal response was observed ($82.2 \pm 3.7\%$ vs. $79.8 \pm 4.1\%$ respectively; methacholine dose response curve before incubation = 100%). Incubation with higher concentrations of MEHP (3.10^{-4} M and 10^{-3} M) resulted in a increased shift of the methacoline dose response curves to the left. A methacholine -log EC_{50} of 5.85 ± 0.08 (3.10^{-4} M) and 6.38 ± 0.05 (10^{-3} M) was found. Moreover a dose dependent reduction of the maximal effect was observed from $79.8 \pm 4.1\%$ (control) to $58.7 \pm 3.8\%$ and $11.3 \pm 0.8\%$ of respectively 3.10^{-4} M and 10^{-3} M MEHP. A concentration of 10^{-6} M H7 induced a decrease in maximal effect of the methacholine dose response curve from $84.6 \pm 2.9\%$ (ethanol incubation) to $61.7 \pm 4.1\%$. However 10^{-6} M H7 did not alter the -log EC_{50} for methacholine (5.28 ± 0.08 compared to the control of 5.34 ± 0.05). After a washing period for 60 min the -log EC_{50} and maximal response for methacholine returned to normal values as measured before incubation, irrespective of the treatment of the trachea. We observed a -log EC_{50} of 5.51 ± 0.09 and an E_{max} of 80.5 ± 2.9 after incubation with 10^{-3} M MEHP and a 60 min washing period.

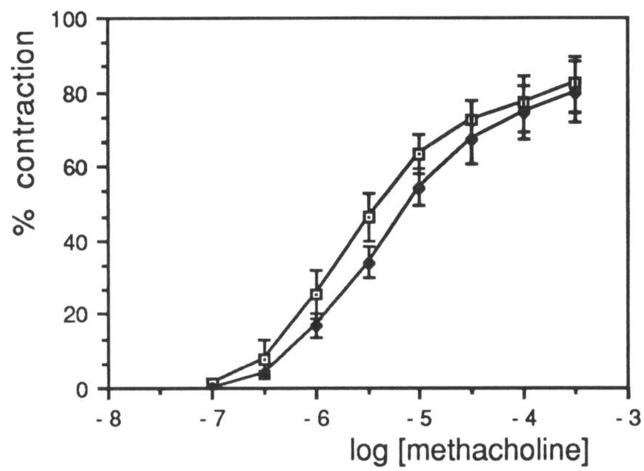

Figure 1: The effect of 10^{-4} M MEHP on methacholine dose response curves of rat tracheal tissue. (♦) control curve and (▫) curve in the presence of 10^{-4} M MEHP.

DISCUSSION

Pulmonary inflammation and increased (non-specific) bronchial reactivity to several stimuli are characteristics of lung diseases like asthma. This clinically observed increased reactivity may be the resultant of either an increase in -log EC_{50} or an increase in maximal response (Ariens, 1987). In the present study we show that the hydrolysis product of DEHP, MEHP induces a dose-dependent increase in -log EC_{50} for methacholine in rat tracheal tissue. However MEHP-incubation also results in a decrease in maximal effect for methacholine. The latter effect is found only at relative high concentrations of MEHP, thus in practive the overall effect of MEHP is the induction of an increased bronchial reactivity to methacholine. The absence of similar effects of DEHP might be explained by its high lipophilicity, rendering it unable to reach its site(s) for action.

The effects of MEHP on the methacholine dose response curve of the rat trachea seem to be reversible. A 60 min. washing period after MEHP incubation results in normal -log EC_{50} and E_{max} values for the methacholine dose response curve. We therefore conclude that only continuous exposure to DEHP might cause bronchial responsiveness and is most dangerous to the lungs.

DEHP and MEHP have been reported to be effective protein kinase C inhibitors (Shukla et al., 1989). The enzyme protein kinase C is involved in the muscarinic receptor transduction pathway (Rang and Dale, 1987). We therefore tested the effects of the known protein kinase C inhibitor H7 on the methacholine dose response curve of the rat trachea. H7 induced a decrease in maximal effect of the muscarinic receptor response but did not influence the -log EC_{50} for methacholine. We thus conclude that the increase in -log EC_{50} after MEHP exposure, is not due to protein kinase C inhibition. Possibly the reduction of the maximal effect for methacholine might be due to inhibition of this enzyme.

The findings of this study are especially relevant to workers in DEHP manufacture and patients recieving multiple blood transfusions. Nevertheless, also the general population could be subject to DEHP/MEHP induced airway hyperreactivity, although the exposure levels are low. It is not unlikely that DEHP/MEHP enhance the bronchial effects of other air pollutants. Inhalation of DEHP/MEHP may aggravate the bronchial hyperresponsiveness in especially patients with CARA.

Acknowledgement:This study is financially supported by the Dutch Asthma Foundation, grant nr 87-30.

REFERENCES:

Ariens, E.J. (1987) Pharmacology of the airway smooth muscle. In: Bronchial hyperresponsiveness (J.A. Nadel, R. Pauwels, R. Snashall, Eds), Blackwell, Oxford, pp. 7-22.

Bennett, S.J., Geelhoed, G.W., Aaron, R.K., Solis, R.T., Hoye, R.C. (1972) Pulmonary injury resulting form perfusion with stored bank blood in the baboon and dog. J. Surg, Res. 13, 295-306.

Bridges, J.W.(1982) Use of toxicity data: a case study of di(2-ethylhexyl)phthalate. In: Toxic hazard assessment of chemicals (M.L. Richardson, Ed), Whitestable, Kent, pp. 233-246.

Doelman, C.J.A., Kramer, K., Timmerman, H., Bast, A. (1988) Vitamin E and selenium regulate balance between beta-adrenergic and muscarinic responses in rat lungs. FEBS Lett 233, 427-431.

Rang, H.P., Dale, M.M. (1987) Pharmacology. Churchill Livingstone, Edinburgh.

Roth, B., Herkenrath, P., Lehmann, H.J. et al. (1988) Di(2-ethylhexyl)phthalate as palsticiser in PVBC respiratory tubing systems: indication of hazardous effects on pulmonary function in mechanically ventilated, perterm infants. Eur. J. Pediatr. 147, 41-46.

Schulz, C.O., Rubin, R.J., Hutchins, G.M. (1975) Acute lung toxicity and sudden death in rats following the intravenous administration of the plasticiser, di(2-ethylhexyl)phthalate, solubilized in Tween surfactants. Toxicol. Appl. Pharmacol. 33, 514-525.

Shukla, R.R., Albro, P.W., Corbett, J.T., Schroeder, J.L. (1989) In vitro studies of the inhibition of protein kinase C from rat brain by di(2-ethylhexyl)phthalate. Chem.-Biol. Interactions 69, 73-85.

Thomas, J.A., Darby, T.D., Wallin, R.F., Garvin, P.J., Martis, L. (1978) A review of the biological effects of di(2-ethylhexyl)phthalate. Toxicol. Appl. Pharmacol. 45, 1-27.

AAS 31:
Mediators in
Airway Hyperreactivity

EICOSANOIDS AND INFLAMMATORY CELLS IN ASTHMA.

Paul M O'Byrne.

The Asthma Research Group, Department of Medicine, McMaster University, Hamilton, Ontario, Canada

INTRODUCTION

Asthma is a common disease, with a cumulative prevalence in many countries of at least 10-15% (Sears, 1990). While dyspnea, wheeze, chest tightness and cough with or without sputum are the usual presenting symptoms in asthma, these symptoms also occur in other conditions and are not specific for asthma. A diagnosis of asthma should be made by objectively documenting reversible airflow obstruction which improves either spontaneously or after treatment. In addition, the presence of airway hyperresponsiveness to a variety of inhaled stimuli is characteristic of asthma (Hargreave et al, 1983). These stimuli include exercise and cold air or chemical bronchoconstrictors, such as histamine or methacholine. In general, patients with more severe airway hyperresponsiveness have more severe asthma, more variable airflow obstruction and require more treatment to control symptoms.

Events occurring in the airways as a result of acute and chronic airway inflammation are important in the pathogenesis of asthma (O'Byrne et al, 1987). This has been known for more than 100 years in patients with severe fatal asthma (Osler,1892). In these patients, a large numbers of inflammatory cells along with epithelial desquamation, mucosal edema and excess secretions are present in the airways (Dunnill et al, 1969). It is now recognized that airway inflammation is also important in milder asthma. For example, studies have demonstrated increases in airway eosinophils and mast cells in patients with very mild, stable asthma (Kirby et al, 1987). The severity of asthma correlates closely with the numbers of these inflammatory cells in the airways. The mechanisms by which airway inflammation may cause airway hyperresponsiveness and airway narrowing in asthma are still largely unknown. It is likely, however, that mediators released from effector cells in the airways cause the influx of inflammatory cells, and subsequent activation of these cells. Further release of mediators from activated cells cause the bronchoconstriction, airway hyperresponsiveness and other manifestations of inflammation such as airway edema and excess airway secretions.

While several mediators have been proposed as playing a role in the pathogenesis of asthma, problems have existed which have prevented convincing evidence being obtained for a role for any mediator. The problems include 1) the difficulties in measuring the mediator or its metabolite at its site of action in the airways; 2) the lack of potent, specific mediator antagonists; 3) the absence of an animal model of asthma. Several animal models of airway hyperresponsiveness exist (Lee et al, 1977; Abraham et al, 1983; Murphy et al, 1986), and studies using these models have lead to interesting and potentially important insights into the pathogenesis of airway hyperresponsiveness. However, definitive studies can only be performed in human subjects, which imposes major limitations on the interventions which can be done to, for example, measure mediator release.

PRODUCTION OF EICOSANOIDS

The release of arachidonic acid from cell membrane phospholipids through the action of a family of phospholipases can result in the production of a wide variety of mediators which may be relevant in the pathogenesis of asthma. These lipid mediators (eicosanoids) have traditionally been considered in two classes: mediators which result from the action of the enzyme cyclooxygenase on arachidonic acid, which are prostaglandins (PGs) or thromboxane (Tx); and mediators which result from the action of the enzyme 5-lipooxygenase on arachidonic acid, which are the leukotrienes (LTs). More recently, however, other products have been identified which result from the activity of different enzymes, such as 12- and 15-lipooxygenase. Lastly, platelet activating factor (PAF) has been recognized to be a mediator derived from arachidonic acid metabolism. This review will focus on the evidence that prostaglandins and thromboxane, and leukotrienes, are released in the airways of asthmatic patients; are responsible for the initiation of airway inflammation; cause bronchoconstriction; and result in the development of airway hyperresponsiveness.

The oxidative metabolism of arachidonic acid by cyclooxygenase produces the cyclic endoperoxides PGG_2 and PGH_2. The subsequent action of prostaglandin isomerases produces either PGD_2 or PGE_2, reductive cleavage produces PGF_{2a}, while one of two terminal synthetases on the endoperoxide produces PGI_2 and TxA_2. Cyclooxygenase appears to be present in most cells; however, the cyclooxygenase metabolite(s) released from a particular cell are quite specific (for example TxA_2 from platelets, and PGI_2 from endothelial cells). This suggests that the terminal synthetases are cell specific.

The effect of 5-lipooxygenase on arachidonic acid is to produce 5-hydroperoxyeicosatetraenoic acid (5-HPETE), which is converted by dehydrase to LTA_4. This intermediate metabolite can be acted upon by epoxide hydrolase resulting in LTB_4, or by glutathione-s-transferase resulting in LTC_4, which is further metabolized to LTD_4 and LTE_4. It is now recognized that the biological activity of previously called slow reacting substance of anaphylaxis (SRS-A) is made up by the sulphidopeptide leukotrienes LTC_4, LTD_4 and LTE_4 (Lewis and Austen, 1984).

PROSTAGLANDINS AND THROMBOXANE

Prostaglandins have a variety of effects on airway function in asthma. They can be most easily be considered in two classes. These are stimulatory prostaglandins, such as PGD_2 and PGF_{2a}, which are potent bronchoconstrictors, and inhibitory prostaglandins, such as PGE_2, which can reduce bronchoconstrictor responses and attenuate the release of bronchoconstrictor mediators, such as acetylcholine, from airway nerves.

Evidence has been obtained in both animal models of airway hyperresponsiveness and in human subjects with asthma that cyclooxygenase metabolites are involved in causing bronchoconstriction and also airway hyperresponsiveness after inhalation of inflammatory stimuli. There is, however, little convincing evidence that cyclooxygenase metabolites are important in causing the ongoing, persisting airway hyperresponsiveness that is characteristic of asthma. This is because several studies have failed to demonstrate any effect of cyclooxygenase inhibitors on stable airway hyperresponsiveness in asthmatic subjects.

The initial studies examining the role of cyclooxygenase metabolites in the pathogenesis of transient airway hyperresponsiveness after an inflammatory stimulus were carried out using the cyclooxygenase inhibitor, indomethacin in dogs with airway hyperresponsiveness after inhaled ozone. Indomethacin did not alter baseline airway responsiveness to inhaled acetylcholine, but did prevent the development of airway hyperresponsiveness after inhaled ozone (O'Byrne et al, 1984). Despite the absence of airway hyperresponsiveness, the magnitude of the inflammatory response, as measured by the numbers of neutrophils in the airway epithelium, was not altered by indomethacin. This suggested that a cyclooxygenase product was not responsible for the chemotaxis of acute inflammatory cells into the airways after inhaled ozone; however, a cyclooxygenase

into the airways after inhaled ozone; however, a cyclooxygenase product was released during the inflammatory response which caused airway hyperresponsiveness. Subsequently, a reputed combined cyclooxygenase and lipooxygenase inhibitor, BW775c was also demonstrated to prevent the development of airway hyperresponsiveness after inhaled ozone in dogs (Fabbri et al, 1985). Inhibition of cyclooxygenase by indomethacin also prevents the development of airway hyperresponsiveness in other species; for example, after C_{5a} des arg in rabbits (Berend et al, 1985), and after inhaled allergen in sheep (Lanes et al, 1986). Other investigators, however, demonstrated that BW775c but not indomethacin, prevents airway hyperresponsiveness after inhaled ozone in guinea pigs (Lee et al, 1985), suggesting that a lipooxygenase rather than a cyclooxygenase product was causing airway hyperresponsiveness in this species.

Cyclooxygenase products have been implicated in the pathogenesis of allergen-induced early asthmatic (Manning et al, 1990) as well as late asthmatic responses (Joubert et al, 1985; Shephard et al, 1985) in human subjects. This has been done by pretreating subjects with several different cyclooxygenase inhibitors. For example, Joubert et al (1985) reported that pretreatment with indomethacin inhibited the late response in 10 out of 11 subjects studied, without having a major effect on the early response. More recent studies, however, have not confirmed these observations on either allergen-induced early or late responses. Pretreatment with indomethacin (100mg/day) did not influence either the early or late asthmatic responses (Kirby et al, 1989). These results suggested that cyclooxygenase products were not important mediators in causing allergen-induced asthmatic responses. There is, however, evidence which implicates a cyclooxygenase product in the pathogenesis of airway hyperresponsiveness in asthmatic subjects. Indomethacin significantly inhibits the development of airway hyperresponsiveness after inhaled allergen in allergic subjects (Kirby et al, 1989). This suggests that a cyclooxygenase product is involved in the pathogenesis of airway hyperresponsiveness after inhaled allergen. The most likely candidates are the stimulatory prostaglandins PGD_2, PGF_{2a} or TxA_2.

STIMULATORY PROSTAGLANDINS

Prostaglandin D_2: PGD_2 is known to be released from stimulated dispersed human lung cells in vitro (Yen and Mathe, 1976) and from the airways of allergic human subjects which have been stimulated by allergen (Murray et al, 1986). PGD_2 is a bronchoconstrictor of human airways (Hardy et al, 1984), and is more potent when inhaled by human subjects than PGF_{2a}. PGD_2 causes bronchoconstriction directly through stimulation of specific contractile receptors and indirectly through acting presynaptically to release acetylcholine from airway cholinergic nerves (Munoz et al, 1986). Subthreshold contractile concentrations of PGD_2 have been demonstrated to increase airway responsiveness to inhaled histamine and methacholine in asthmatic subjects (Fuller et al, 1986). Thus, PGD_2 released in human airways after allergen inhalation has the potential to both cause acute bronchoconstriction and increase airway hyperresponsiveness to other constrictor mediators. However, selective receptor antagonists for PGD_2 or inhibitors of its production are not available to allow a precise evaluation of the importance of this cyclooxygenase metabolite in causing asthmatic responses.

Prostaglandin F_{2a}: As with PGD_2, PGF_{2a} has the potential for being important in causing bronchoconstriction and airway hyperresponsiveness after inhaled allergen in human subjects. This is because is released from human lungs, is a potent bronchoconstrictor in asthmatic airways (Thomson et al, 1981), and inhaled subthreshold constrictor concentrations can increase airway responsiveness in dogs (O'Byrne et al, 1984) and human subjects (Fish et al, 1984). As with PGD_2, there are no selective PGF_{2a} receptor antagonists available, which would allow identification of the importance of these metabolites in causing these responses. Indeed, it has been suggested that all contractile prostaglandins act via a single TP_1-receptor (Gardiner, 1989). Therefore, differentiation of the relative importance of the contractile prostaglandins in causing asthmatic responses may prove to be extremely difficult.

Thromboxane A_2: TxA_2 is a potent constrictor of smooth muscle. TxA_2 was originally described as being released from platelets (Hamberg et al, 1975), but is now known to be released from other cells, including macrophages and neutrophils (Higgs et al, 1983). The biological half-life of TxA_2 is very short (approximately 30s); therefore implicating TxA_2 in disease processes has depended on measurement of its more stable metabolite Thromboxane B_2 (TxB_2) in biological fluids; on the use of the stable endoperoxides U44069 or U46619, which mimic most of the biological effects of TxA_2 and have been used as TxA_2 analogs; and on the use of inhibitors of TxA_2 synthesis and antagonists of the TxA_2 receptor. Using these techniques, TxA_2 has been implicated in the pathogenesis of airway hyperresponsiveness in dogs (Aizawa et al, 1985) and primates (McFarlane et al 1988); of the late cutaneous response to intradermal allergen (Dorsch et al, 1983) in humans; of the immediate response to inhaled allergen in dogs (Kleeberger et al, 1987); of the late asthmatic response after inhaled allergen in humans (Sherherd et al, 1985); and of airway hyperresponsiveness in asthmatic subjects (Fujimura et al, 1986).

The mechanism by which TxA_2 causes airway hyperresponsiveness is not yet known, but possible mechanisms include presynaptic modulation of acetylcholine release, or an effect on airway smooth muscle. TxA_2 was demonstrated to modulate acetylcholine release in airways initially by Munoz et al (1986). No increase in the responses to exogenous acetylcholine was demonstrated, suggesting that the augmentation was occurring presynaptically, through increased acetylcholine release in response to field stimulation. Further support for this hypothesis was provided by Tamaoki et al (1987), who demonstrated that aggregated platelets in an organ bath released TxA_2, which transiently increased the responses to field stimulation and this effect was prevented by a TxA_2 receptor antagonist. Once again, the responses to an exogenous cholinergic agonist was not altered by the released TxA_2.

Attempts to measure TxB_2 in human subjects during asthmatic episodes or following allergen challenge have lead to conflicting results. Joubert et al (1985) and Manning et al (1990) have demonstrated increased levels of TxB_2 in plasma following allergen challenge. However, plasma TxB_2 measurements must be viewed with caution because of the possibility of local platelet generation of TxB_2 and measurements should be confirmed by assaying the 2,3-dinor metabolite of TxB_2 which cannot come from platelet activation alone.

The TxA_2 synthetase inhibitor, OKY 046, administered orally, reduces acetylcholine airway hyperresponsiveness in stable asthmatic subjects (although these studies were uncontrolled), while a lipooxygenase inhibitor had no effect in these subjects (Fujimura et al 1986). Thus, TxA_2 may be an important mediator in the pathogenesis of airway hyperresponsiveness either in stable asthma or after inhaled allergens. Recent studies, however, have examined the effect of the thromboxane synthetase inhibitor, CGS 13080, on airway responses after allergen challenge. CGS 13080 slightly but significantly inhibited the magnitude of the early but not the late responses after inhaled allergen. In addition, there was no effect on airway hyperresponsiveness to inhaled histamine measured at 24h post allergen (Manning et al, 1990).

These studies taken together, suggest that thromboxane may be released following allergen challenge, and be partly responsible for the early asthmatic response, but in contrast to dogs, is not important in causing airway hyperresponsiveness following allergen inhalation.

INHIBITORY PROSTAGLANDINS

While the differentiation of the prostaglandins into stimulatory and inhibitory classes is somewhat inappropriate, the main action of PGE_2 and PGI_2 on airway function is to relax airway smooth muscle and to antagonize the contractile responses of other bronchoconstrictor agonists.

The evidence that inhibitory prostaglandins play a role in modulating the contractile responses of agonists such as histamine and acetylcholine comes from studies which have demonstrated that tachyphylaxis (a decreased response to repeated stimulation) occurs following repeated challenges with exercise or inhaled histamine in asthmatic subjects, when challenges are separated by up to 6 hr (O'Byrne and Jones, 1986; Manning et al, 1987) . In addition, both exercise refractoriness and histamine tachyphylaxis are prevented by pretreatment with indomethacin (O'Byrne and Jones, 1986; Manning et al, 1987), which suggests that tachyphylaxis occurs through release of inhibitory prostaglandins in the airways. Lastly pretreatment of asthmatic subjects with oral PGE_1, in doses which do not cause bronchodilation, reduce airway responsiveness to both histamine and methacholine (Manning et al, 1989). These results are consistent with studies of airway smooth muscle <u>in vitro</u>, where histamine tachyphylaxis occurs through inhibitory prostaglandin release (Anderson et al, 1977), and with studies in dogs <u>in vivo</u> where histamine tachyphylaxis is inhibited by indomethacin (Shore and Martin, 1985). In addition, histamine tachyphylaxis in asthmatic subjects is blocked by pretreatment with cimetidine in asthmatics (Jackson et al, 1988), suggesting that H_2 receptor stimulation is involved with the development of histamine tachyphylaxis. Stimulation of H_2 receptors in the lung in vitro has previously been shown to be associated with PGE_2 release in guinea-pigs (Yen and Mathe, 1976), and PGE_2 release from canine trachealis by histamine is antagonized by cimetidine (Manning et al, 1988).

Contraction of asthmatic airways by histamine also reduces airway responsiveness to acetylcholine (Manning and O'Byrne, 1988) and exercise (Hamilec et al, 1988). This lack of specificity suggests that either receptor downregulation or an alteration of the contractile properties of airway smooth muscle is occurring. Indeed, PGE causes heterologous receptor desensitization in some isolated cell systems and airway smooth muscle has specific PGE receptors (Gardiner, 1989) mediating inhibitory effects such as relaxation. However, there is no current evidence from either in vivo or in vitro preparations to support this speculation.

SULPHIDOPEPTIDE LEUKOTRIENES

The importance of slow reacting substance of anaphylaxis (SRS-A) in the events occurring after immunological challenge of the lungs was identified in the early 1940's (Kellaway and Trethewie 1940). Later, Brocklehurst demonstrated that SRS-A was released from lung segments from an asthmatic subject, when these segments were exposed to allergen (1960). SRS-A was suggested to be an important mediator in causing symptoms after exposure to allergen in sensitized subjects, mainly because it was a potent airway smooth muscle constrictor with a much longer duration of action than other smooth muscle constrictors, such as histamine. SRS-A is now known to consist of the sulphidopeptide leukotrienes (LT) C_4, D_4 and E_4 (Lewis and Austen, 1984). Thus, there is evidence that the sulphidopeptide leukotrienes are released from a number of cells present in the airways, including mast cells, which are involved in the airway responses to inhaled allergen (Dahlen et al,

1983). Also, the leukotrienes have potent effects on human airway smooth muscle (Dahlen et al, 1980), and inhaled LTC_4 and LTD_4 are potent bronchoconstrictors in both normal and asthmatic subjects (Adelroth et al, 1986), being up to 10,000 times more potent than methacholine in some normal subjects (Griffin et al, 1983), with a longer duration of action than inhaled histamine (Barnes et al, 1984).

Sensitized sheep develop both an early and late bronchoconstrictor response after inhalation of ascaris suum antigen. Pretreatment of these sheep with a leukotriene antagonist FPL 55712 abolished the late response after both inhaled allergen (Lanes et al, 1986) and compound 48/80, a non-immunological stimulus for mast cell degranulation (Russi et al, 1984). This suggests that a leukotriene, presumably released from mast cells, is responsible for the late response. Subsequently, Abraham et al (1985) demonstrated that inhaled LTD_4 caused both an early and late response in the allergic sheep. These observations have led these investigators to suggest that LTD_4, released as part of the early response, initiates a series of events which leads to the late response. Several investigators have demonstrated that urinary LTE_4 increases during the early response after inhaled allergen in human subjects (Manning et al, 1989; Taylor et al, 1989), but not during the late response (Manning et al, 1989). Also, inhalation of LTD_4 by atopic asthmatic subjects who develop a late response after allergen inhalation, in concentrations sufficient to cause bronchoconstriction of similar magnitude to the early response after inhaled allergen, does not cause a late response (Higgins et al, 1987). Therefore in human subjects, release of LTD_4 during the early response after inhaled allergen is not, by itself, sufficient to cause a late asthmatic response. However, the precise role of LTC_4 or D_4 in the asthmatic responses after inhaled allergen is not yet clarified.

There is some evidence that the sulphidopeptide leukotrienes cause airway hyperresponsiveness in asthmatic

with LTE_4 (1984) increased responsiveness of guinea-pig tracheal strips to histamine. Kern et al (1986) have demonstrated that precontraction of airways with LTD_4 in normal subjects will increase airway responsiveness to inhaled methacholine. Also, Barnes et al (1984) reported that inhaled LTD_4 increased airway responsiveness to prostaglandin F2a, but not to histamine. The time course of this effect of LTD_4 is not known. Also, Lee et al (1987) demonstrated that inhaled LTE_4 transiently increased airway responsiveness to inhaled histamine. Lastly, Bel et al (1987) have reported that pretreatment with LTD_4 increased the maximal bronchoconstrictor response achieved by inhaled methacholine, and this effect lasted for 3 days. Therefore, the evidence collected to date would support a role for the sulphidopeptide leukotrienes in the pathogenesis of airway hyperresponsiveness after stimuli such as allergen; however, their precise role in these responses awaits studies using a specific receptor antagonist.

The chemotactic leukotriene B_4 (LTB_4) may also be important in causing airway hyperresponsiveness. Holtzman et al (1983) have demonstrated that isolated canine tracheal epithelial cells produced LTB_4 when stimulated with arachidonate. In addition, human alveolar macrophages, known to be present in airway lumen, produce more LTB_4 than almost any other cell (Lewis and Austen, 1984). These data raised the possibility that the potent chemotactic LTB_4 may be responsible for initiating inflammatory response after stimuli such as allergen. Subsequently, inhaled LTB_4 was demonstrated to cause influx of neutrophils into canine airways and the development of airway hyperresponsiveness (O'Byrne et al, 1985). However, inhaled LTB_4 does not cause airway hyperresponsiveness when inhaled by human subjects (Black et al, 1989).

CONCLUSIONS

There is now convincing evidence that eicosaniods are released from inflammatory cells and perhaps some structural cells in human airways, and are important in both causing and modulating bronchoconstrictor responses in asthmatic subjects. It is much less clear whether eicosaniods are involved in causing either airway inflammation or airway hyperresponsiveness, which are such characteristic features of asthma. The final proof will depend on studies using potent and selective antagonists for these mediators and examining the effects of these antagonists on bronchoconstrictor responses, airway hyperresponsiveness and airway inflammation in asthmatic subjects.

REFERENCES

Abraham WM, Delehunt JC, Yerger L, Marchette B. Characterization of a late phase pulmonary response after antigen challenge in allergic sheep. Am Rev Respir Dis 1983; 128:839-844.

Abraham WM, Russi E, Wanner A, Delehunt JC, Yerger LD, Chapman GA. Production of early and late pulmonary responses with inhaled leukotriene D_4 in allergic sheep. Prostaglandins 1985; 29:715-727.

Adelroth E, Morris MM, Hargreave FE, O'Byrne PM. Airway responsiveness to leukotrienes C4 and D4 and to methacholine in patients with asthma and normal controls. N Engl J Med 1986; 315:480-484.

Aizawa H, Chung KF, Leikauf GD, Ueki I, Bethel RA, O'Byrne PM, Hirose T, Nadel JA. Significance of thromboxane generation in ozone-induced airway hyperresponsiveness in dogs. J Appl Physiol 1985; 59:1918-1923.

Anderson WH, Krzanowski JJ, Polson JB, Szentivanyi A. Characteristics of histamine tachyphylaxis in canine tracheal smooth muscle. Naunyn-Schiedeberg Arch Pharmacol 1977;308:117 -125.

Barnes NC, Piper PJ, Costello JF. Comparative effects of inhaled leukotriene C4, leukotriene D4 and histamine in normal human subjects. Thorax 1984;39:500-04.

Barnes NC, Watson A, Koulouris N, Piper PJ, Costello J. Effect of preinhalation of leukotriene D4 on sensitivity to prostaglandin F2a. Thorax 1984;39:697.

Bel EH, van der Veen H, Kramps JA, Dijkman JH, Sterk PJ.

Maximal airway narrowing to inhaled leukotriene D4 in normal subjects: comparison and interaction with methacholine. Am Rev Respir Dis 1987; 136:979-84.
Berend N, Armour CL, Black JL. Indomethacin inhibits C5a des arg-induced airway hyperresponsiveness in the rabbit. Am Rev Respir Dis 1985;131:24A.
Black PN, Fuller RW, Taylor GW, Barnes PJ, Dollery CT. Effect of inhaled leukotriene B_4 alone and in combination with prostaglandin D_2 on bronchial responsiveness to histamine in normal subjects. Thorax 1989; 44:491-5.
Brocklehurst WE. The release of histamine and formation of a slow-recacting substance (SRS-A) during anaphylatic shock. J Physiol 1960;151:416-35.
Dahlen SE, Hansson G, Hedqvist P, Bjorck T, Gramstrom E, Dahlen B. Allergen challange of lung tissue from asthmatics elicts bronchial contraction that correlates with the release of leukotrienes C4, D4 and E4. Proc Natl Acad Sci USA 1983; 80:1712-16.
Dahlen SE, Hedqvist P, Hammarstrom S, Samuelsson B. Leukotrienes are potent constrictors of human bronchi. Nature 1980;288:484-86.
Dorsch WD, Ring J, Melzer H. A selective inhibitor of thromboxane biosynthesis enhances immediate and inhibits late cutaneous allergic reactions in man. J Allergy Clin Immunol 1983; 72:168-174.
Dunnill MS, Massarell GR, Anderson JA. A comparison of the quantitive anatomy of the bronchi in normal subjects, in status asthmaticus, in chronic bronchitis and in emphysema. Thorax 1969;24:176-79.
Fabbri LM, Aizawa H, O'Byrne PM, Bethel RA, Walters EH, Nadel JA, Holtzman MJ. An anti-inflammatory drug (BW755c) inhibits airway responsiveness induced by ozone in dogs. J Allergy Clin Immunol 1985;76:162-6.
Fish JE, Jameson A, Albright A, Norman PS. Modulation of bronchomoter effects of chemical mediators by PGF2a. Amer Rev Respir Dis 1984;129:A2.
Fujimura M, Sasaki F, Nakatsumi Y, Takahashi Y, Hifumi S, Taga K, Mifune J-I, Tanaka T, Matsuda T. Effects of a thromboxane synthetase inhibitor (OKY-046) and a lipoxygenase inhibitor (AA-861) on bronchial responsiveness to acetylcholine in asthmatic subjects. Thorax 1986; 41:955-59.
Fuller RW, Dixon CMS, Dollery CT, Barnes PJ. Prostaglandin D_2 potentiates airway responsiveness to histamine and methacholine. Am Rev Respir Dis 1986;133:252-54.
Gardiner PJ. Eicosanoids and airway smooth muscle. Pharm Ther 1989; 44:1-62.
Griffin M, Weiss JW, Leitch AG, McFadden ER, Corey EJ, Austen KF, Drazen JM. Effects of leukotriene D4 on the airways in asthma. N Engl J Med 1983; 308:436-439.
Hamberg M, Svensson J, Samuelsson B. Thromboxanes: a new group of biologically active compounds derived from prostaglandin endoperoxides. Proc Natl Acad Sci USA 1975; 72:2994-8.

Hamilec CM, Manning PJ, O'Byrne PM. Exercise refractoriness post histamine bronchoconstriction in asthmatic subjects. Am Rev Respir Dis 1988; 138:794-98.
Hardy CC, Robinson C, Tattersfield AE, Holgate ST. The bronchoconstrictor effect of inhaled prostaglandin D_2 in normal and asthmatic men. N Engl J Med 1984;311:209-13.
Hargreave FE, Ryan G, Thomson NC, O'Byrne PM, Latimer K, Juniper EF, Dolovich J. Bronchial responsiveness to histamine or methacholine in asthma: measurement and clinical significance. J Allergy Clin Immunol 1981; 68:347-355.
Higgins DA, O'Byrne PM. Inhaled leukotriene D4 does not cause a late response in atopic subjects. J Allergy Clin Immunol 1987;79:141A.
Higgs GA, Moncada S, Salmon JA, Seager K. The source of thromboxane and prostaglandins in experimental inflammation. Br J Pharmac 1983; 79:863-68.
Holtzman MJ, Aizawa H, Nadel JA, Goetzl EJ. Selective generation of leukotriene B4 by tracheal epithelial cells from dogs. Biochem Biophys Res Commun 1983;114:1071-76.
Jackson PA, Manning PJ, O'Byrne PM. A new role for histamine H_2-receptors in asthmatic airways. Am Rev Respir Dis 1988; 138:784-88.
Joubert JR, Shephard E, Mouton W, Van Zyk L, Viljoen I. Non -steroid anti-inflammatory drugs in asthma: dangerous or useful therapy? Allergy 1985;40:202-207.
Kellaway CH, Trethewie ER. The liberation of a slow-reacting smooth muscle-stimulating substance in anaphylaxis. Q J Exp Physiol 1940;30:121-45.
Kern R, Smith LJ, Patterson R, Krell RD, Bernstein PR. Characterization of the airway responses to inhaled leukotriene D4 in normal subjects. Am Rev Respir Dis 1986;133:1124-26.
Kleeberger SR, Kolbe J, Adkinson NF Jr, Peters SP, Spannhake EW. Thromboxane contributes to the immediate antigenic response of canine peripheral airways. J Appl Physiol 1987; 62:1589-95.
Kirby JG, Hargreave FE, Cockcroft DW, O'Byrne PM. The effect of indomethacin on allergen-induced asthmatic responses. J Appl Physiol 1989; 66:578-83.
Kirby JG, Hargreave FE, Gleich GJ, O'Byrne PM. Bronchoalveolar cell profiles of asthmatic and nonasthmatic subjects. Am Rev Respir Dis 1987; 136:379-83.
Lanes S, Stevenson JS, Codias E, Hernandez A. Sialczak MW, Wanner A, Abraham WM. Indomethacin and FPL 55321 inhibit antigen-induced airway hyperresponsiveness in sheep. J Appl Physiol 1986;61:864-72.
Lee HK, Murlas C. Ozone-induced bronchial hyperreactivity in guinea pigs is abolished by BW 755C or FPL 55712 but not by indomethacin. Am Rev Respir Dis 1985; 132:1005-1009.
Lee L-Y, Bleeker ER, Nadel JA. Effect of ozone on bronchomotor response to inhaled histamine in dogs. J Appl Physiol 1977; 43:626-31.

Lee TH, Arm JP, Spur BW. Leukotriene E4 (LTE4) enhances airways histamine responsiveness in asthmatic subjects. J Allergy Clin Immunol 1987;79:256A.

Lee TH, Austen KF, Corey EJ, Drazen JM. Leukotriene E_4-induced airway hyperresponsiveness of guinea pig trachea smooth muscle to histamine and evidence for three seperate sulfidopeptide leukotriene receptors. Proc Natl Acad Sci USA 1984:81;4922-4925.

Lewis RA, Austen KF. The biologically active leukotrienes. Biosynthesis, metabolism, receptors, functions and pharmachology. J Clin Invest 1984;73:889-97.

Manning PM, Jones GL, Lane CG, O'Byrne PM. Histamine-induced prostaglandin E_2 release from canine tracheal smooth muscle is inhibited by H_2-receptor blockade. Am Rev Respir Dis 1988; 137:373A.

Manning PJ, Jones GL, O'Byrne PM. Tachyphylaxis to inhaled histamine in asthmatic subjects. J Appl Physiol 1987; 63:1572-77.

Manning PJ, Lane CG, O'Byrne PM. The effect of oral prostaglandin E_1 on airway responsiveness in asthmatic subjects. Pulmonary Pharmacology 1989: 1989; 2:121-24.

Manning PJ, O'Byrne PM. Histamine bronchoconstriction reduces airway responsiveness in asthmatic subjects. Am Rev Respir Dis 1988; 137:1323-25.

Manning PJ, Rokach J, Malo JL, Ethier D, Cartier A, Girard Y, Charleson S, O'Byrne PM. Urinary leukotriene E_4 levels during early and late asthmatic responses. Am Rev Respir Dis 1989; 139:A92

Manning PJ, Stevens WH, Cockcroft DW, O'Byrne PM. The role of thromboxane in allergen-induced asthmatic responses. Am Rev Respir Dis 1990; 141:A395.

McFarlane CS, Ford-Hutchinson AW, Letts LG. Inhibition of thromboxane (TxA_2)-induced airway hyperresponsiveness to aerosolized acetylcholine by the selective TxA_2 antagonist L655,240 in the conscious primate. Am Rev Respir Dis 1988; 137:100A.

Munoz NM, Shioya T, Murphy TM, Primack S, Dame C, Sands MF, Leff AR. Potentiation of vagal contractile response by thromboxane mimetic U-46619. J Appl Physiol 1986; 61:1173-9.

Murray JJ, Tonnel AB, Brash AR, Roberts LJ, Gosset P, Workman R, Capron A, Oates JA. Release of prostaglandin D_2 into human airways during acute antigen challenge. N Engl J Med 1986; 315:800-4.

Murphy KR, Wilson MC, Irvin CG, Glezen LS, Marsh WR, Haslett C, Henson PM, Larsen GL. The requirement for polymorphonuclear leukocytes in the asthmatic response and heightened airways reactivity in an asthmatic model. Am Rev Respir Dis 1986; 134:62-68.

O'Byrne PM, Aizawa H, Bethel RA, Chung KF, Nadel JA, Holtzman MJ. Prostaglandin F2a increases airway responsiveness of pulmonary airways in dogs. Prostaglandins 1984;28:537-43.

O'Byrne PM, Jones GL. The effect of indomethacin on exercise -induced bronchoconstriction and refractoriness after exercise. Am Rev Respir Dis 1986; 134:69-72.
O'Byrne PM, Kirby JG, Hargreave FE. Airway inflammation and hyperresponsiveness. Am Rev Respir Dis 1987; 136:S35-S37.
O'Byrne PM, Leikauf GD, Aizawa H, Bethel RA, Ueki IF, Holtzman MJ, Nadel JA. Leukotriene B4 induced airway hyperresponsiveness in dogs. J Appl Physiol 1985;59:1941-1946.
O'Byrne PM, Walters EH, Aizawa H, Fabbri LM, Holtzman MJ, Nadel JA. Indomethacin inhibits the airway hyperresponsiveness but not the neutrophil influx induced by ozone in dogs. Am Rev Respir Dis 1984: 130:220-224.
Osler W. In: The Principals and Practice of Medicine. Appleton and Co., New York, NY. 1892:497.
Russi AW, Perruchoud AP, Yerger LD, Stevenson JS, Tabak J, Marchette B, Abraham WM. Late phase bronchial obstruction following nonimmunologic mast cell degranulation. J Appl Physiol 1984; 57:1182-1188.
Sears MR. Epidemiology of Asthma (1990). In: Asthma as an Inflammatory Disease. New York, Marcel Dekker, Inc, 1-34.
Shephard EG, Malan L, Macfarlane CM, Mouton W, Joubert JR. Lung function and plasma levels of thromboxane B_2, 6 -ketoprostaglandin F_{1a} and B-thromboglobulin in antigen-induced asthma before and after indomethacin pretreatment. Br J Clin Pharm 1985; 19:459-470.
Shore S, Martin JG. Tachyphylaxis to inhaled aerosolized histamine in anesthetized dogs. J Appl Physiol 1985; 59:1355 -1363.
Tamaoki J, Sekizawa K, Osborne ML, Ueki IF, Graf PD, Nadel JA. Platelet aggregation increases cholinergic neurotransmission in canine airway. J Appl Physiol 1987; 62:2246-51.
Taylor GW, Black P, Turner N, Taylor I, Maltby NH, Fuller RW, Dollery CT. Urinary leukotriene E_4 after antigen challenge and in acute asthma and allergic rhinitis. Lancet 1989; i:584-87.
Thomson NC, Roberts R, Bandouvakis J, Newball H, Hargreave FE. Comparison of bronchial responses to prostaglandin F2a and methacholine. J Allergy Clin Immunol 1981;68:392-8.
Yen SS, Mathe AA, Dugan JJ. Release of prostaglandins from healthy and sensitized guinea-pig lung and trachea by histamine. Prostaglandins 1976; 11:227-39.

AAS 31:
Mediators in
Airway Hyperreactivity

THE EFFECT OF PROSTANOIDS ON THE FUNCTION OF HUMAN EOSINOPHILS

P.R. Butchers and C.J. Vardey

Department of Peripheral Pharmacology, Glaxo Group Research Ltd., Ware, Hertfordshire, U.K.

SUMMARY: The effects of prostanoids on eosinophil cationic protein (ECP) release and eosinophil migration have been measured. ECP release was inhibited by prostanoids active on DP and EP receptors. In contrast the DP agonist protaglandin D_2 enhanced eosinophil migration.

INTRODUCTION

Inflammation in the lungs of allergic asthmatics is characterized by an infiltration of eosinophils (De Monchy et al., 1985). Eosinophils are capable of releasing a range of noxious agents, including major basic proteins and cationic proteins, which probably contribute to local tissue damage and exacerbation of inflammation (Filley et al., 1982; Gleich et al., 1983). The factors that control eosinophil activation, migration and degranulation under these conditions have not, however, been clearly defined.

It is likely that prostanoids are released during inflammation in the lungs. Sensitized mast cells produce prostaglandin (PG) D_2 on contact with allergen (Schleimer et al., 1984), and increases in PGD_2 have been measured in bronchoalveolar lavage fluid of asthmatics challenged with allergen (Murray et al., 1986). Invading leucocytes, such as neutrophils and eosinophils (Goldstein et al., 1977; Hubscher, 1975), and resident cells such as alveolar macrophages (MacDermot, 1984) are also capable of synthesizing prostanoids. Little work has been performed, however, to investigate whether prostanoids influence eosinophil function.

In these studies, we have evaluated a series of natural and synthetic prostanoids on two aspects of human eosinophil function: the release of eosinophil cationic protein (ECP) and eosinophil migration.

MATERIALS

The materials used were obtained from the following sources:- Percoll, Ficoll-Paque and eosinophil cationic protein (ECP) radioimmunoassay from Pharmacia, U.K.; formyl-methionyl-leucyl-phenylalanine (FMLP), zymosan and cytochalasin B from Sigma, U.K.; cetyltrimethylammonium bromide (CTAB) from Aldrich, U.K.; plasmagel from Roger Bellon Labs, France; microchemotaxis chamber from Neuroprobe, USA; polycarbonate filters from Nucleopore, USA; Prostaglandins E_2 and $F_{2\alpha}$ were obtained from Upjohn, U.K.; Cicaprost from Schering AG, West Germany; U46619 from Cayman Chemicals, USA. Misoprostol was a gift from G.D. Searle, USA and BW245C a gift from Burroughs-Wellcome, U.K. PGD_2 and sulprostone were synthesized at Glaxo Group Research Ltd., Ware, U.K.

Zymosan-activated serum (ZAS) was prepared by incubating pre-boiled zymosan at a concentration of 5mg/ml in human serum for 1hr at 37^oC. The zymosan was centrifuged and the supernatant ZAS removed and stored at $^-20^oC$.

METHODS

Isolation of Granulocytes: Venous blood was drawn from the forearm of healthy human volunteers and anti-coagulated with 10 IU heparin/ml blood. The blood was mixed with 0.67 times volume of plasmagel and left to sediment at 37^oC for 35-40 min. The supernatant buffy coat was removed by aspiration, underlayed with a half volume of Ficoll-Paque and centrifuged at 400g for 20 min at 22^oC. The granulocyte pellet was washed twice in calcium-free tris buffer, NaCl, 122mM; KCl, 2.7mM; Tris, 25mM; Glucose, 5.6mM; $MgCl_2$, 1.0mM; BSA, 0.1% w/v, pH 7.4, washed again in tris buffer containing $CaCl_2$, 1mM and then resuspended in buffer. An aliquot of the final suspension was stained with chromotrope 2R and the eosinophils counted in an improved Neubauer counting chamber. Granulocyte populations contained a minimum of 2% eosinophils (mean 6.7%). The remaining cells were almost exclusively neutrophils.

In all studies, indomethacin (3µM) and adenosine deaminase (1U/ml) were incorporated into the buffer to inhibit the endogenous production of prostaglandins and remove any adenosine released by the cells.

<u>Eosinophil Cationic Protein Release</u>: Eosinophil cationic protein (ECP) release was used as a marker for degranulation. Cytochalasin B (10µM) was incorporated into the buffer to enhance the amount of ECP released on challenge with FMLP (0.2µM). Granulocytes were resuspended to $5x10^4$ eosinophils/ml and aliquots (200µl) were warmed to 37°C, prior to the addition of prostanoid or vehicle (25µl). After a further 10 min, the cells were challenged with FMLP or vehicle (25µl) and incubated for a further 10 min at 37°C. The granulocyte suspension was centrifuged and the supernatant collected into CTAB (final concentration 0.2%) and assayed for ECP by radioimmunoassay.

<u>Eosinophil Migration</u>: The effect of prostanoids on eosinophil migration to ZAS (diluted 1 in 20 in buffer) was measured using a 48-well microchemotaxis chamber with a 3µm pore polycarbonate filter. Granulocytes were resuspended to $5x10^6$ cells/ml and 50µl of the suspension was placed above the filter. ZAS or buffer (25µl) was placed below the filter. Prostanoids were incorporated into the buffer both above and below the filter. The chamber was then incubated for 2hr at 37°C. The upper half of the chamber, together with filter and gasket were removed and the granulocytes in the lower chamber stained and counted for eosinophils.

RESULTS

Eosinophil Cationic Protein Release: Upon stimulation with FMLP (0.2μM), the granulocyte suspensions released 1.2 ± 0.2μg ECP/10^6 eosinophils (mean ± sem; n=18). The natural prostaglandins, PGD_2, PGE_2 and to a lesser extent, $PGF_{2\alpha}$ inhibited ECP release, although the inhibitory effects were only apparent at concentrations of 1.0μM and above (Figure 1). The maximum inhibition obtained varied between blood donors, and was frequently less than 50%. The synthetic analogues of PGI_2 (cicaprost; 0.01-1.0μM) and thromboxane A_2 (U46619; 0.01-10.0μM) showed no inhibitory activity.

The most potent prostanoid was the selective DP receptor agonist, BW245C. Although the inhibition curve was shallow and only achieved a maximum of 40%, BW245C was at least an order of magnitude more potent than PGD_2 (Figure 2). The EP_2/EP_3 receptor agonist, misoprostol showed a similar profile to PGE_2, whereas the EP_1/EP_3 receptor agonist, sulprostone was inactive (Figure 3).

Eosinophil Migration: PGD_2 (0.1-10μM) enhanced the migration of eosinophils to zymosan-activated serum (ZAS), the most significant response ($p<0.01$) being seen at 1.0μM PGD_2 (Figure 4). However, in the absence of ZAS, PGD_2 at 1.0 and 10.0μM stimulated migration in its own right. In contrast, PGE_2, $PGF_{2\alpha}$ and U46619 (0.1-10μM) failed to influence the migration of eosinophils to ZAS.

DISCUSSION

Studies on prostanoids has led to a classification of receptor subtypes based upon the activities of natural and synthetic agonists and antagonists (Coleman et al., 1990). In this study, we have investigated the effects of prostanoids on two aspects of human eosinophil function, and have attempted to identify the receptors involved. The data indicate that

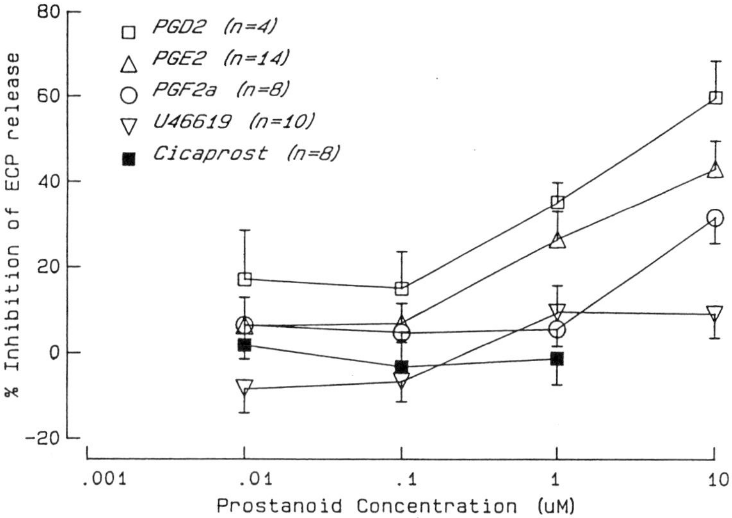

Figure 1

The effect of Prostanoids on Eosinophil Cationic Protein release from Human Granulocytes
Points are means ± sem of n experiments

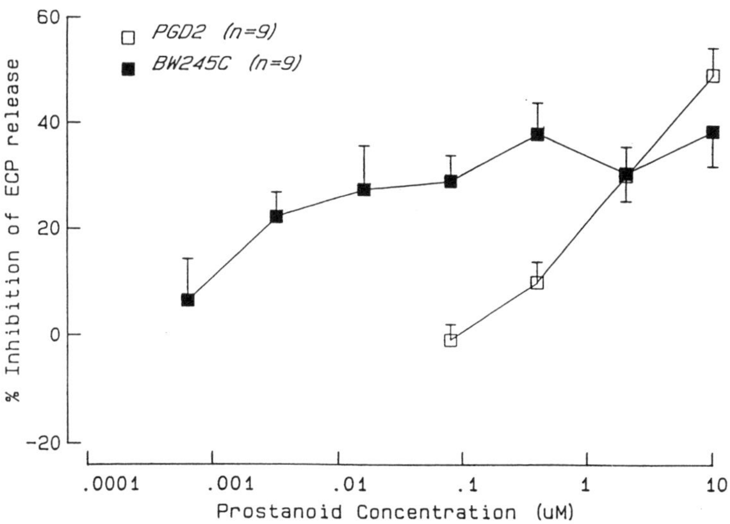

Figure 2

The effect of DP-selective Prostanoid agonists on Eosinophil Cationic Protein release from Human Granulocytes
Points are means ± sem of n experiments

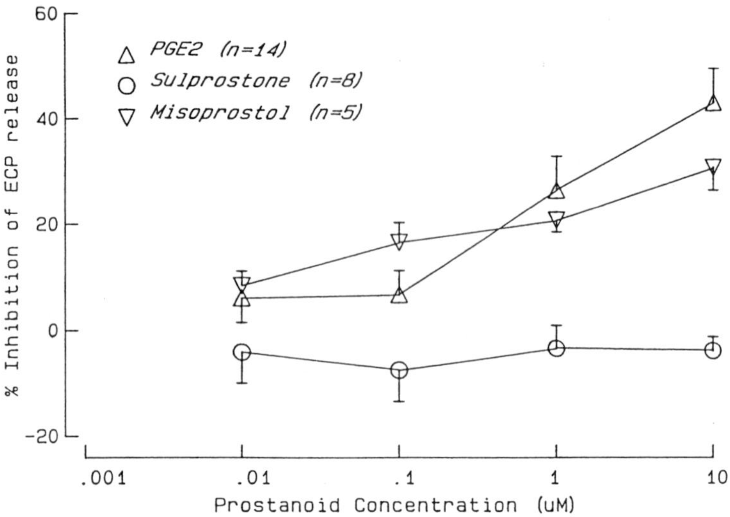

Figure 3

The effect of EP-selective Prostanoid agonists on Eosinophil Cationic Protein release from Human Granulocytes Points are means ± sem of n experiments

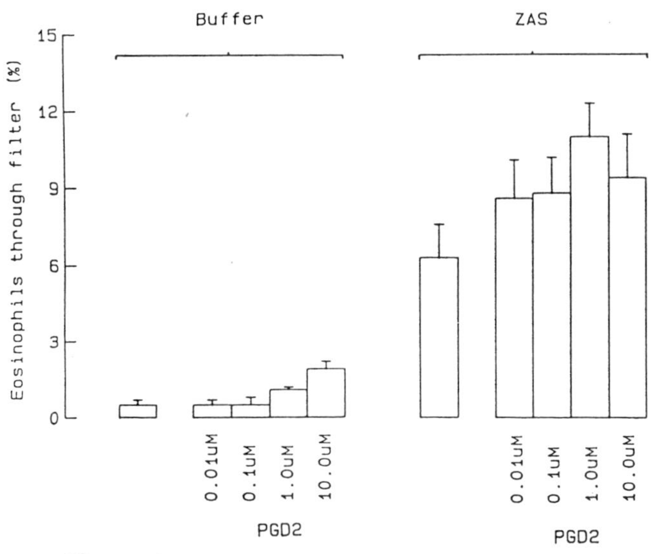

Figure 4

The effect of Prostaglandin D2 on Eosinophil Migration Bars are means ± sem of 7 experiments

prostanoids can have both inhibitory and stimulatory effects on this cell type.

Eosinophil cationic protein (ECP) is one of four toxic basic proteins released by the eosinophil. It is contained within the matrix of the specific granule and may be released selectively on stimulation (Khalife et al., 1986). In this study, ECP release was stimulated using the bacterial peptide, FMLP. Other workers have shown FMLP to stimulate leukotriene release from eosinophils (Shaw et al., 1985) and to enhance eosinophil cytotoxic activity (Kay et al., 1987).

The natural prostaglandins, PGD_2, PGE_2 and $PGF_{2\alpha}$ showed weak inhibitory effects on FMLP-induced ECP release. The potencies of the DP-receptor agonists, PGD_2 and BW245C, both in absolute terms and relative to one another were similar to those seen on other DP-receptor containing preparations, such as human platelets (Keery & Lumley, 1988; Narumiya & Toda, 1985) where the compounds cause inhibition of aggregation.

The potency of PGE_2 was less than that previously reported on a range of EP-receptor containing preparations, notably smooth muscle (Dong et al., 1986). However, the inhibitory effects of the EP_2/EP_3-receptor agonist, misoprostol and the lack of effect of the EP_1/EP_3 receptor agonist, sulprostone suggest that inhibition may be mediated by the EP_2-receptor subtype.

In using a mixed granulocyte population, there is the possibility of an interaction between neutrophil products and eosinophils. This may be important since neutrophils have been reported to have inhibitory prostanoid receptors (Zurier et al., 1974). Studies are therefore underway to evaluate the effects of prostanoids on a purified human eosinophil population. Initial results indicate that DP- and EP-receptor agonists are able to inhibit ECP release from purified (>70%) eosinophils (P. Butchers, unpublished observations).

The relevance of leucocyte migration in vitro to the accumulation of cells at an inflammatory site in vivo is the subject of much controversy (Spry, 1988). It is likely, however, that some leucocyte movement is required, if only to traverse the endothelial cell barrier. The chemokinetic effects of PGD_2 have previously been described by Goetzl and co-workers (1979) using purified eosinophils from a patient with chronic active hepatitis. The data presented here show similar effects of PGD_2 on normal human eosinophils, albeit at higher concentrations. Whether the receptor is of the same subtype as that causing inhibition of ECP release is under investigation. It is interesting to note that increases in PGD_2 have been measured in the lungs of asthmatics challenged with allergen (Murray et al., 1986), and that PGD_2 has been shown to reduce circulating eosinophils (Marsden et al., 1984) and to increase eosinophils in the tracheal lumen of dogs (Emery et al., 1989).

In conclusion, our studies have shown that prostanoids, specifically those active at DP- and EP-receptors, have modulatory effects on the function of normal human eosinophils. However, these effects require relatively high concentrations of the natural agonists, and may reflect low receptor numbers on these cells. Whether such concentrations of prostanoids occur locally in vivo, or whether eosinophil sensitivity to these autocoids changes in disease states, is at present unclear.

REFERENCES

Coleman, R.A., Kennedy, I., Humphrey, P.P.A., Bunce, K. & Lumley, P. (1990). Prostanoids and their receptors. In: Comprehensive Medicinal Chemistry Vol. 3, Membranes and their Receptors (C. Hansch, P.G. Sammes and J.B. Taylor, Eds), Pergamon Press, Oxford, pp 643-706.

DeMonchy, J.G., Kauffman, H.F., Venge, P., Koeter, G.H., Jansen, H.M., Sluiter, H.J. & DeVries, K. (1985). Bronchoalveolar eosinophilia during allergen-induced late asthmatic reactions. Am. Rev. Respir. Dis. 131, 373-376.

Dong, Y.J., Jones, R.L. & Wilson, N.H. (1986). Prostaglandin E receptor subtypes in smooth muscle: Agonist activities of stable prostacyclin analogues. Br. J. Pharmacol. 87, 97-107.

Emery, D.L., Djokic, T.D., Graf, P.D. & Nadel, J.A. (1989). Prostaglandin D_2 causes accumulation of eosinophils in the lumen of the dog trachea. J. Appl. Physiol. 67, 959-962.

Filley, W.V., Holley, K.E., Kephart, G.M. & Gleich, G.J. (1982). Identification by immunofluorescence of eosinophil granule major basic protein in lung tissues of patients with bronchial asthma. Lancet 2, 11-16.

Gleich, G.J., Loegering, D.A., Frigas, E. & Filley, W.V. (1983). The eosinophil granule major basic protein: Biological activities and relationship to bronchial astham. Monogr. Allergy 18, 237-83.

Goetzl, E.J., Weller, P.F. & Valone, F.M. (1979). Biochemical and functional bases of the regulatory and protective roles the human eosinophil. In: Advances in Inflammation Research (G. Weissman, Ed), Raven Press, New York, pp 157-167.

Goldstein, I.M., Malmstem, C.L., Samuelsson, B. and Weissman, G. (1977). Prostaglandins, thromboxanes and polymorphonuclear leukocytes: mediation and modulation of inflammation. Inflammation 2, 309-317.

Hubscher, T. (1975). Role of the eosinophil in the allergic reactions. II. Release of prostaglandins from human eosinophilic leukocytes. J. Immunol. 114, 1389-1393.

Kay, A.B., Walsh, G.M., Moqbel, R., Macdonald, A.J., Nagakura, T., Carroll, M.P. & Richerson, H.B. (1987). Disodium cromoglycate inhibits activation of human inflammatory cells in vitro. J. Allergy. Clin. Immunol. 80, 1-8.

Keery, R.J. & Lumley, P. (1988). AH6809, a prostaglandin DP-receptor blocking drug on human platelets. Br. J. Pharmacol. 94, 745-754.

Khalife, J., Capron, M., Cesbron, J.Y., Tai, P-C., Taelman, H., Prin, L. & Capron, A. (1986). Role of specific IgE antibodies in peroxidase (EPO) release from human eosinophils. J. Immunol. 137, 1659-1664.

MacDermot, J., Kelsey, C.R., Waddell, K.A., Richmond, R., Knight, R.K., Cole, P.J., Dollery, C.T., Landon, D.N. & Blair I.A. (1984). Synthesis of leukotriene B_4 and prostanoids by human alveolar macrophages analysed by gas chromatography/mass spectrometry. Prostaglandins 27, 163-179.

Marsden, K.A., Rao, P.S., Cavanagh, D. & Spaziani, E. (1984). The effect of prostaglandin D_2 (PGD_2) on circulating eosinophils. Prostaglandins, Leukotrienes Med., 15, 387-397.

Murray, J.J., Tonnel, A.B., Brash, A.R., Roberts, L.J., Gosset, P., Workman, M.D., Capron, A. & Oates, J.A. (1986). Release of prostaglandin D_2 into human airways during acute antigen challenge. N. Engl. J. Med. 315, 800-804.

Narumiya, S.R. & Toda, N. (1985). Different responsiveness of prostaglandin D_2-sensitive systems to prostaglandin D_2 and its analogues. Br. J. Pharmacol., 85, 367-375.

Schleimer, R.P., MacGlashen, D.W., Peters, S.P., Naderio, R., Proud, D., Adkinson, N.F. & Lichtenstein, L.M. (1984). Inflammatory mediators and mechansims of release from purified human basophils and mast cells. J. Allergy. Clin. Immunol., 74, 473-481.

Shaw, R.J., Walsh, G.M., Cromwell, O., Moqbel, R., Spry, C.J. & Kay, A.B. (1985). Activated human eosinophils generate SRS-A leukotrienes following IgG-dependent stimulation. Nature, 316, 150-152.

Spry, C.J.F. (1988). In: Eosinophils. A comprehensive review and guide to the scientific and medical literature. Oxford University Press, pp 95-102.

Zurier, R.B., Weissmann, G. Hoffstein, S., Kammerman, S. and Tai, H.H. (1974). Mechanisms of lysosomal enzyme release from human leukocytes. II. Effects of cAMP and cGMP, autonomic antagonists, and agents which effect microtubule function. J. Clin. Invest. 53, 297-309.

MODULATION OF GUINEA PIG AIRWAY REACTIVITY BY THE LINOLEIC ACID METABOLITE 13-HYDROXY-OCTADECADIENOIC ACID (13-HODE).

F. Engels, P.A.J. Henricks, H.J. van der Linde and F.P. Nijkamp

Department of Pharmacology, Faculty of Pharmacy, University of Utrecht, Catharijnesingel 60, 3511 GH Utrecht, The Netherlands.

SUMMARY: The influence of the linoleic acid metabolite 13-hydroxy-octadecadienoic acid (13-HODE) on guinea pig tracheal reactivity to both contractile and relaxant agonists was investigated *in vitro*. 13-HODE induced an increased contraction of tracheal rings to histamine, whereas methacholine responsiveness was not significantly affected. Relaxant responses to isoprenaline and prostaglandin E_2 were not influenced either.

Pulmonary epithelial cells play an important role in airway smooth muscle function. Epithelial cells produce lipid mediators, including hydroxy metabolites of linoleic acid (Henricks et al., 1990a), which may be involved in the regulation of smooth muscle function. These mediators are also produced by inflammatory cells, which are abundant at pulmonary sites of inflammation. In the present studies we investigated the influence of 13-hydroxy-octadecadienoic acid (13-HODE) on guinea pig tracheal reactivity.

MATERIALS AND METHODS

Dunkin-Hartley guinea pigs were killed by an overdose of pentobarbital sodium i.p. Tracheas were taken and cut into rings, which were suspended in organ baths and connected to isometric transducers (Harvard Bioscience). The experimental protocol included: (1) a 15 min phase during which 4 g tension was applied to the tracheal preparations, followed by a change to 2 g tension, (2) a 60 min equilibration period during which the medium was refreshed 3 times, (3) a 30 min incubation with 10 µM 13-HODE, and (4) a dose-response curve to cumulative concentrations of agonists.

13(S)-HODE was purchased from Oxford Biomedical Research, Inc., Oxford (MI), U.S.A. All other reagents were of analytical grade.

RESULTS

Incubation of guinea pig tracheal rings with 10 µM 13-HODE for 30 min resulted in a statistically significant increase of maximal contraction to histamine (see table I). The EC_{50} values of the dose-response curves did not differ. In contrast, contraction to the cholinergic muscarinic agonist methacholine was not significantly affected. Relaxant responses to isoprenaline or prostaglandin E_2 (PGE_2), which were measured after a submaximal precontraction with methacholine, were also not influenced by 13-HODE.

DISCUSSION

Fatty acid derived mediators, including prostaglandins, leukotrienes and monohydroxy derivatives of arachidonic acid (HETEs), have a wealth of biological activities which play a role in physiology and pathophysiology of airway function (Wasserman, 1986; Krell & Snyder, 1987). Derivatives of linoleic acid may be equally important in this respect, as the hydroxy derivatives (HODEs) are formed by various cell types in the lungs (Engels et al., 1986, 1990; Oosthuizen et al., 1990).

TABLE I. The influence of 13-HODE (10 μM) on the reactivity of guinea pig tracheal rings to various contractile and relaxant agonists.

	maximum response (mgf)	-log EC_{50} (M)
Histamine:		
- 13-HODE	1044 ± 327	5.38 ± 0.10
+ 13-HODE	1642 ± 119*	5.30 ± 0.15
Methacholine:		
- 13-HODE	2315 ± 174	6.10 ± 0.07
+ 13-HODE	2819 ± 296	5.99 ± 0.08
Isoprenaline:		
- 13-HODE	2188 ± 322	6.97 ± 0.07
+ 13-HODE	2340 ± 275	7.01 ± 0.07
Prostaglandin E_2:		
- 13-HODE	2487 ± 328	6.84 ± 0.16
+ 13-HODE	2232 ± 133	6.80 ± 0.10

*Statistically significant at $P < 0.05$
Data are presented as mean ± S.E.M. of 6-9 individual experiments.

We have previously shown that HODEs influence inflammatory cell activity in the airways, i.e. HODEs display a modulatory activity towards reactive oxygen species from guinea pig pulmonary macrophages (Engels et al., 1989). In addition, HODEs possess chemotactic activity for bovine and human polymorphonuclear leukocytes (Henricks et al., 1990b). Since bronchial hyperresponsiveness is often associated with inflammatory reactions in the airways (Chung & Barnes, 1987), linoleic acid metabolites may affect airway function via their effects on inflammatory cells. In the present communication we present evidence that HODEs may also directly affect airway smooth muscle function. Thus, 13-HODE induced a hyperresponsiveness of isolated tracheal segments of the guinea pig for histamine. This effect was rather specific, as methacholine, isoprenaline, and prostaglandin E_2 reactivity were not changed. The mechanism whereby histamine reactivity is enhanced is not yet known. Data from Henry et al. (1987) suggest that 9-HODE can increase basal adenylate cyclase activity in platelet membranes. However, bronchial smooth muscle contraction to histamine is mediated by H_1 receptors (Joad & Casale, 1987), which are coupled to the hydrolysis of inositol phospholipids, and not to adenylate cyclase. Further research will have to clarify this issue.

Acknowledgement: These studies were financially supported by the Dutch Asthma Foundation (grant 86.17).

REFERENCES

Chung, K.F. and Barnes, P.J. (1987) Bronchial hyperresponsiveness and inflammation in asthma. In: Asthma Reviews (J. Morley, ed.), Academic Press, London, pp. 25-41.

Engels, F., Willems, H. and Nijkamp, F.P. (1986) Cyclooxygenase catalyzed formation of 9-hydroxy linoleic acid by guinea pig alveolar macrophages under non-stimulated conditions. FEBS Letters 209, 249-253.

Engels, F., Henricks, P.A.J., van der Vliet, H. and Nijkamp, F.P. (1989) Modulatory activity of 9-hydroxy- and 9-hydroperoxy-octadecadienoic acid towards reactive oxygen species from guinea-pig pulmonary macrophages. Eur. J. Biochem. 184, 197-203.

Engels, F., Drijver, A.A. and Nijkamp, F.P. (1990) Modulation of the release of 9-hydroxy-octadecadienoic acid and other fatty acid derived mediators from guinea-pig pulmonary macrophages. Int. J. Immunopharmac. 12, 199-205.

Henricks, P.A.J., Engels, F., van Esch, B., van der Linde, H.J., Oosthuizen, M.J. and Nijkamp, F.P. (1990a) Epithelium-derived linoleic acid metabolites modulate airway smooth muscle function. In: Mediators in Airway Hyperreactivity. Agents and Actions Supplement (F.P. Nijkamp, F. Engels, P.A.J. Henricks,

A.J.M. van Oosterhout, eds.), Birkhäuser Verlag, Basel, pp. 283-286.

Henricks, P.A.J., Engels, F., van der Vliet, H. and Nijkamp, F.P. (1990b) 9- and 13-hydroxy-linoleic acid possess chemotactic activity for bovine and human polymorphonuclear leukocytes. Submitted for publication.

Henry, D.Y., Gueritte-Voegelein, F., Insel, P.A., Ferry, N., Bouguet, J., Potier, P., Sevenet, T. and Hanoune, J. (1987) Isolation and characterization of 9-hydroxy-10-trans,12-cis-octadecadienoic acid, a novel regulator of platelet adenylate cyclase from Glechoma hederacea L. Labiatae. Eur. J. Biochem. 170, 389-394.

Joad, J.P. and Casale, T.B. (1987) Airway histamine H_1 receptors. In: Current Topics in Pulmonary Pharmacology and Toxicology, Vol. 3 (M.A. Hollinger, ed.), Elsevier Science Publishing Co., Inc., New York, pp. 95-121.

Krell, R.D. and Snyder, D.W. (1987) Pulmonary physiology, pharmacology, and biochemistry of the leukotrienes. In: Current Topics in Pulmonary Pharmacology and Toxicology, Vol. 3 (M.A. Hollinger, ed.), Elsevier Science Publishing Co., Inc., New York, pp. 174-209.

Oosthuizen, M.J., Engels, F., van Esch, B., Henricks, P.A.J. and Nijkamp, F.P. (1990) Production of arachidonic and linoleic acid metabolites by guinea pig tracheal epithelial cells. Inflammation 14, 401-408.

Wasserman, M.A. (1986) Bronchopulmonary effects of arachidonic acid metabolites. In: Current Topics in Pulmonary Pharmacology and Toxicology, Vol. 1 (M.A. Hollinger, ed.), Elsevier Science Publishing Co., Inc., New York, pp. 1-22.

AAS 31:
Mediators in
Airway Hyperreactivity

THE EFFECT OF DRUGS ON LUNG HYPERREACTIVITY IN SEPHADEX TREATED RATS

B.A.Spicer R.C.Baker and H.Smith

SmithKline Beecham Pharmaceuticals, Biosciences Research Centre, Epsom, Surrey KT18 5XQ, U.K.

SUMMARY: The injection of Sephadex G200 intravenously into rats induced a blood eosinophilia and an hyper-reactivity of lung parenchymal strips to 5-hydroxytryptamine (5HT) and carbachol. The blood eosinophilia and the hyper-reactivity to 5HT reached a maximum at the same time and before that to carbachol. It was shown previously that the reduction of the blood eosinophilia by treatment with dexamethasone, dapsone, phenidone, isoprenaline and aminophylline also reduced the hyper-reactivity to 5HT. In this study we found that only dexamethasone reduced the hyper-reactivity to carbachol.

Asthma is associated with an increased responsiveness of the airways to inhaled bronchoconstrictor agents such as methacholine. The hyper-responsiveness can be reduced by the administration of glucocorticosteroids but restoration to normal is rarely achieved. Few studies have been carried out comparing the responsiveness of lung tissue from asthmatics and normals and results have been inconclusive [Whicker, *et al.*,(1988) DeJongste, *et al.*,(1987)]. Asthma is also associated with an eosinophilia in the blood and bronchoalveolar lavage (BAL) fluid. The role of the eosinophil in asthma is still not clear but it is thought to be involved in the development of the hyper-responsiveness [Taylor, *et al.*, (1987)]. The injection of Sephadex G200 intravenously into rats induced a blood eosinophilia and an hyper-responsiveness of the lungs which can be measured both *in vivo* and *in vitro*. This model has been used to identify compounds which affect either the number of eosinophils or the hyper-responsiveness [Spicer, *et al.*, (1990)].

MATERIALS AND METHODS

Methods

Sephadex G200, was suspended in isotonic saline at 0.5mg/ml and stored at 4°C for 48h. 1ml of the suspension was injected intravenously into Charles Rivers Sprague Dawley rats, 250-350g, on days 0, 2 and 5. Rats in a control group received saline. Drugs were given before each injection of Sephadex either subcutaneously as freshly made neutral solution in isotonic saline or orally as solutions or suspensions in 0.5% methylcellulose. 20μl samples of blood, taken from the tail vein of the rats, were added to 10ml of Isoton II, and total cell counts determined using a Coulter Counter Model DN. Differential leucocyte counts were carried out by fixing and staining a blood smear with May-Grunwald and Giemsa stains.

Rats were stunned and bled and the heart and lungs removed and placed in a modified Tyrode's solution at room temperature. The initial 2 to 3mm of the left lobe was removed and then two consecutive strips were cut at right angles to the bronchus 3 to 4mm wide. The lung strip was suspended in 4ml organ baths which contained oxygenated modified Tyrode's solution at 37°C. The response of the tissue was recorded isometrically. A tension of 1gm was applied to the tissue and the tissue was allowed to stabilise for one hour. During this time the bathing fluid was changed by upward displacement at 15 minute intervals and the tension restored after each wash. Cumulative dose-response curves of the parenchymal lung strips to 5HT were obtained. The tissues were allowed to recover over a 30 minute period with washing at 15 minute intervals. A cumulative dose response curve to carbachol was then obtained. The areas under the dose response curve were calculated.

RESULTS

Injection of Sephadex G200 intravenously into rats on days 0, 2 and 5 induced a hyper-responsiveness in the lungs to carbachol. (Figure 1). There was a marked increase in the reactivity of the tissue to carbachol as shown by an increase in the slope of the dose-response curve. There was little change in the sensitivity as measured by ED_{50} dose, that is the dose required to produce a response of 50% of its own maximum. A similar increase in reactivity was obtained for 5HT [Spicer, *et al.*,(1990)]. The time course for the development of the hyper-reactivity to 5HT and carbachol differ. The hyper-reactivity which developed to 5HT and the increase in the number of eosinophils reached a maximum on day 7.

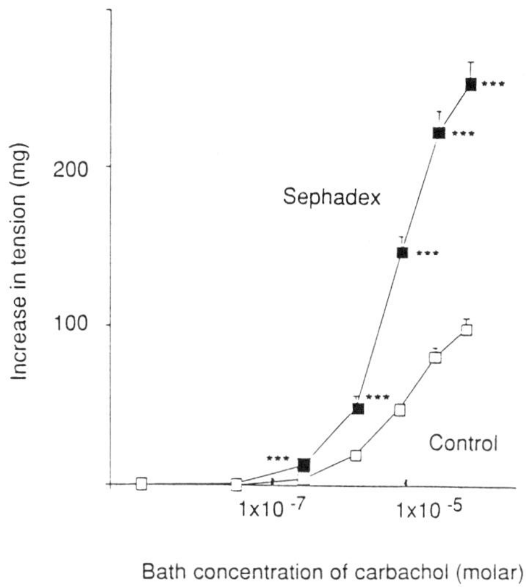

Fig 1: Effect of injecting Sephadex G200 intravenously into rats on days 0,2 and 5 on the responsiveness of lung strips to carbachol ■ on day 8 compared with lung strips from naive rats □ Results are Mean ± SEM n > 10; **p - < 0.01; *** p - < 0.001 compared to naive animals.

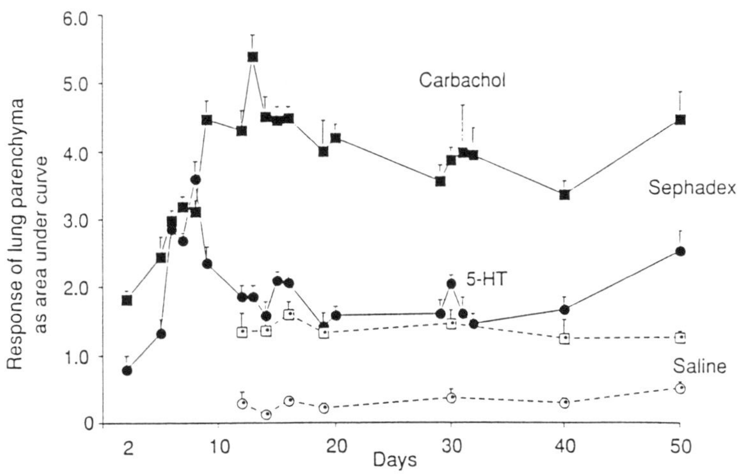

Fig 2: Response of lung parenchymal strips taken from rats given Sephadex G200 on day 0. 2 and 5 to 5HT ■ or carbachol • compared with the response in saline treated rats to 5HT □ or carbachol ○ Results are Means ± SEM n > 10. Responses of Sephadex treated rats were significantly different (p - < 0.001) from saline treated rats except on day 2.

The blood eosinophilia returned to control levels by day 20 but the hyper-reactivity to 5HT was still present at 40 days, although at a reduced level. The hyper-reactivity to carbachol reached a maximum on day 12 and remained at this level for at least 40 days. (Figure 2)

Drugs were given to the rats before each injection of Sephadex at doses at which they were known to reduce the blood eosinophilia on day 7: dexamethasone (0.1mg/kg p.o. 4 hours), dapsone (100mg/kg p.o. 30 mins), phenidone (100mg/kg p.o. 30 mins), isoprenaline (0.1mg/kg s.c. 10 mins), aminophylline (100mg/kg p.o. 30 mins). Of these drugs only dexamethasone reduced the hyper-reactivity to carbachol from $100 \pm 4\%$ to $69 \pm 8\%$ as area under the dose-response curve (n>10; p-<0.01) on days 6, 7 and 8.

DISCUSSION

The injection of Sephadex G200 intravenously into rats induced a blood eosinophilia and an hyper-reactivity to 5HT and carbachol. It was shown previously that drugs which inhibited the blood eosinophilia also inhibited the hyper-reactivity to 5HT and there was a marked correlation between blood eosinophil numbers and the hyper-reactivity to 5HT [Spicer, *et al.*, (1990)]. In this study we found that the time course for the development of the hyper-reactivity to 5HT and the eosinophilia were similar. These data show that the development of the hyper-reactivity to 5HT is closely associated with the eosinophilia. In contrast reduction of the eosinophilia with drugs, with the exception of dexamethasone, had no effect on the hyper-reactivity to carbachol. The increase in reactivity to carbachol reached a maximum after the eosinophilia had peaked and persisted when the eosinophil numbers had returned to normal. The hyper-reactivity to carbachol was not directly associated with the eosinophilia.

REFERENCES

Whicker,S.D.,Armour,C.L.,Black,J.L.(1988). Responsiveness of bronchial smooth muscle from asthmatic patients to relaxant and contractile agents. Pulmonary Pharm.1,25-31.

De Jongste,J.C.,Mans,H.,Bouta,I.L.,Kerrebijn,K.F.(1987). In vitro responses of airways from an asthmatic patient. Eur.J.Resp.Dis.71,23-29.

Taylor,K.J.,Luksza,A.R. (1987). Peripheral blood eosinophil counts and bronchial responsiveness. Thorax 42, 452-456.

Spicer,B.A.,Baker,R.C.,Laycock,S.M.,Smith,H. (1990). The effects of drugs on Sephadex induced eosinophilia and lung hyper-responsiveness in the rat.Brit.J.Pharm.(submitted).

AAS 31:
Mediators in
Airway Hyperreactivity

ADENYL CYCLASE ACTIVITY IN HUMAN ALVEOLAR MACROPHAGES

F.D. Beusenberg[1], J.G.C. van Amsterdam[1], J.M.E. van Schaik[1], H.C. Hoogsteden[2] and I.L. Bonta[1]

Departments of Pharmacology[1] and Pulmonary Medicine[2], Erasmus University Rotterdam[1] and University Hospital Dijkzigt[2], Post Office Box 1738, 3000 DR, Rotterdam, The Netherlands.

SUMMARY

The inflammatory mediators PGE_2, DC-PGI_2 and histamine as well as the ß-adrenergic drugs isoprenaline and salbutamol increase intracellular cyclic AMP-concentrations whereas Platelet Activating Factor does not induce any change in adenyl cyclase activity of normal human alveolar macrophages. Functional H_2-histaminergic and $ß_2$-adrenergic receptor-subtypes are coupled to macrophage adenyl cyclase.

INTRODUCTION

During the last few years substantial experimental evidence has been raised for the involvement of inflammation in the development of bronchial hyperresponsiviness, one of the most pronounced features of asthma and chronic obstructive pulmonary diseases (COPD). Many different inflammatory cells, like mast cells, eosinophils but predominantly alveolar macrophages, release mediators which interact in a complex way to induce inflammation-related changes in the airways (Barnes et al., 1988). In these pathological conditions, macrophages act, through their specific and non- specific characteristics (e.g. phagocytosis, activation of the immunological response, and the production of a variety of mediators), as modulators of the inflammatory process (Rankin, 1989). In turn, these mediators modulate the activity of alveolar macrophages through receptor-mediated mechanisms. These cellular functions are closely related to the intracellular concentrations of a second messenger, cyclic AMP. Increases in intracellular cyclic AMP-concentrations are generally reflected with a down-regulation of cellular activity.

In the presented study, we examined the effects of some inflammatory mediators known to be involved in the pathophysiology of asthma and COPD (prostaglandin E_2, prostacyclin, histamine and platelet activating factor) and frequently used anti-athmatic drugs, the beta-adrenergic agonists isoprenaline and salbutamol on the adenyl cyclase activity in human alveolar macrophages (AM) of normal healthy smoking and subjects.

MATERIALS AND METHODS

Subjects

The study included 29 healthy smoking (n=25), male (n=4) and female (n=25) volunteers. Mean age was 34 ± 9.4 years. All subjects did not receive any medication during three weeks prior to Broncho Alveolar Lavage (BAL) and had no history of pulmonary disorders.

Broncho Alveolar Lavage

BAL was performed after premedication with thiazinaminum and local anesthesia using a lidocaine 2 percent spray. The bronchoscope was placed in wedge position in the right middle lobe, and four volumes of 50 ml sterile saline solution was infused and aspirated immediately in a siliconized specimen trap placed on melting ice.

Cell-isolation, -purification and -incubation

Alveolar macrophages were purified by a Ficoll-Isopaque (Nycomed, Oslo, Norway) gradient centrifugation procedure after which the cells were washed and incubated for 15 min. in the presence of IBMX (a phosphodiesterase-inhibitor by Janssen Chimica, Beerse, Belgium) and the inflammatory mediators prostaglandin E_2 (PGE_2), prostacyclin ($DC\text{-}PGI_2$, a stable analogue), histamine or platelet activating factor (PAF) or the beta-adrenergic drugs isoprenaline or salbutamol. When used, the selective histaminergic antagonists mepyramine and cimetidine and the adrenergic antagonist propranolol, were added to the sellsuspensions on ice, 5 min. prior to incubation (10 μM). After the incubationperiod, cells were disrupted and intracellular cyclic AMP- concentrations were determined by a high-affinity protein binding method (Bonta et al., 1984).

RESULTS

Table 1 summerizes the agonist-induced cyclic AMP- increases in human alveolar macrophages of healthy smoking subjects.

	-log[concentration] (M)				
agonist	**8**	**7**	**6**	**5**	**4**
PGE2	132 ± 13	213 ± 18	351 ± 42	479 ± 61	
DC-PGI2	110 ± 7	141 ± 13	202 ± 32	331 ± 52	
Histamine	106 ± 3	118 ± 7	159 ± 28	183 ± 31	215 ± 35
+ mepyramine	104 ± 4	105 ± 3	114 ± 10	127 ± 27	185 ± 14
+ cimetidine	103 ± 0	101 ± 2[(a)]	105 ± 3[(b)]	106 ± 3[(b)]	103 ± 3[(b)]
PAF[(c)]	100 ± 6	101 ± 7	101 ± 3	105 ± 10	100 ± 2
Isoprenaline	123 ± 12	196 ± 21	252 ± 31	275 ± 36	
+ propranolol	97 ± 1	100 ± 3[(b)]	97 ± 3[(b)]	100 ± 5[(b)]	100 ± 3[(b)]
Salbutamol	102 ± 3	115 ± 4	149 ± 6	165 ± 9	176 ± 10
+ propranolol	100 ± 2	93 ± 3[(a)]	92 ± 4[(b)]	97 ± 3[(b)]	100 ± 4[(b)]

Table 1: Cyclic AMP- concentrations in response to agonist-exposure; incubationprocedure as described in materials and methods; Data expressed as percentage of basal value (basal value = 100 %);a:$P<0.05$, b:$P<0.01$ as compared to data obtained with vehicle alone; c: dose range of 10^{-13}-10^{-9} M did not induce any change in cyclic AMP- concentration.

The inflammatory mediators PGE_2, $DC\text{-}PGI_2$ and histamine induce a dose-dependent increase in intracellular cyclic AMP-levels whereas PAF does not induce any change of adenyl cyclase activity.

Both the beta-adrenergic drugs isoprenaline and salbutamol stimulate adenyl cyclase, however salbutamol, as compared to the full agonist isoprenaline, acts as a partial agonist.

Furthermore, using selective receptor-antagonists, it was shown that histamine, isoprenaline and salbutamol exert their effects on adenyl cyclase activity through H_2-histaminergic resp. Beta$_2$-adrenergic receptors.

DISCUSSION AND CONCLUSIONS

In this study we examined the effects of inflammatory mediators known to be related to the pathophysiology of asthma and COPD and some ß-adrenergic drugs on the adenyl cyclase activity of human alveolar macrophages. PGE_2, DC-PGI_2 and histamine induced a dose-dependent increase in intracellular cyclic AMP-concentrations whereas platelet activating factor does not induce any change in adenyl cyclase activity in human alveolar macrophages (dose-range from 10^{-13}-10^{-5} M). Furthermore, the ß-adrenergic drugs isoprenaline (full agonist) and salbutamol (partial agonist) also enhance cyclic AMP-concentrations. In addition, using selective receptor-antagonists, it was shown that functional H_2-histaminergic and $ß_2$-adrenergic receptors are coupled to macrophage adenyl cyclase.
We conclude that mediators and frequently used anti-asthmatic drugs (like salbutamol and anti-histaminics) have, besides their benificial action on bronchial smooth muscles, an important reducing effect on the activity of alveolar macrophages.

Financially supported by the Dutch Asthma Foundation (NAF).

REFERENCES

Barnes, P.J., Chung, F.K., Page C.P.(1988) Inflammatory mediators and asthma. Pharmacological Rev., 40, 49-84.

Bonta I.L., Adolfs M.J.P., Fieren M.W.J.A. (1984) Cyclic AMP levels and their regulation by prostaglandins in peritoneal macrophages af rats and humans.In : Advances in Cyclic Nucleotide and Protein Phosphorylation Research 17, 615-620. ed. P. Greengard et al.

Rankin, J.A. (1989) The contribution of alveolar macrophages to hyperreactive airway disease. J. Allergy Clin. Immunol. 83, 722-729.

AAS 31:
Mediators in
Airway Hyperreactivity

ACTIVATED HUMAN GRANULOCYTES CONTRACT ISOLATED HUMAN AIRWAYS

R.C. Jongejan, J.C. de Jongste, H.C. Raatgeep, I.L. Bonta and K.F. Kerrebijn

Department of Pediatrics, Subdivision of Pediatric Respiratory Medicine, and Department of Pharmacology, Erasmus University / Sophia Children's Hospital, 3038 GE Rotterdam, The Netherlands.

SUMMARY: Human granulocytes activated with serum treated zymosan (0.2 mg/ml) contract isolated human airways. The magnitude of the contraction depends on the number of granulocytes and the proportion of eosinophils among the granulocytes. The contraction is blocked by a leukotriene C_4/D_4 (LTC_4/D_4) receptor antagonist and by inhibition of lipoxygenase. This suggests that eosinophils rather than neutrophils are implicated in this response, which seems to be caused by LTC_4/D_4.

In atopic asthmatics inhalation of allergen causes an early bronchoconstriction which may be followed by a late broncho-obstructive phase (Booij-Noord et al., 1972). During this late asthmatic reaction (LAR) there is an influx of inflammatory cells into the airway wall (Beasley et al., 1989). Increased numbers of eosinophils and neutrophils have been found in bronchial lavage fluid obtained 6 - 48 hours after allergen challenge (De Monchy et al., 1985). Therefore we investigated the effect of activated human granulocytes on isolated human airways.

MATERIALS AND METHODS

Bronchial rings were dissected from human lung tissue obtained at thoracotomy for lung cancer as described previously (Jongejan et al., 1988). In short, non-cartilaginous bronchi (Ø 1-2 mm)

were identified, cannulated, cleaned from adherent tissue and cut into segments of 3-4 mm length which were stored overnight in a slow flow of cold Krebs-Henseleit buffer. The next day the segments were mounted between two small polished stainless steel hooks and placed in siliconized 10 ml organ baths. The preparations contracted against an isotonic load of 250 mg and were stimulated twice with methacholine (10^{-5}M, 10^{-4}M) before the experiments.

Granulocytes were isolated according to the method by Yazdanbakhsh et al. (1985). Briefly, heparinized blood from healthy volunteers was diluted with phosphate buffered saline (pH 7.4) containing trisodium citrate and centrifuged at room temperature over a Ficoll-Metrizoate gradient of 1.077 g/ml density. Erythrocytes in the pellet were lysed by repeated incubation with ice-cold isotonic ammoniumchloride. Total cell number was counted in a Bürker cell chamber and viability was tested with the trypan blue exclusion test. Differential counts were obtained after staining according to May-Grünwald/Giemsa.

To study the effect of granulocytes on the contractile state of the preparations 1, 2, 5, 10, or 20×10^6 granulocytes were added to the bath. Time-parallel controls received no granulocytes. Next, the cells were activated by adding serum-treated zymosan (STZ, 0.2 mg/ml), which was followed by contraction.

To elucidate if eicosanoids or histamine contributed to the bronchoconstriction evoked by STZ-activated granulocytes, aliquots of 0.5 ml containing 10×10^6 granulocytes were incubated for 15 minutes with either the lipoxygenase inhibitor nordihydroguaiaretic acid (NDGA 10 µM), the LTC_4/D_4 receptor antagonist FPL 55712 (11.5 µM), the cyclo-oxygenase inhibitor indomethacin (10 µM) or the histamine-receptor antagonist mepyramine (2.8 µM), and added to the organ bath. The bronchial rings in the bath that received the cells had simultaneously been incubated with the same drug as the cells. For control preparations and granulocyte suspensions the same procedure was followed but without a drug. Contractions were expressed as a percentage of the maximal response to methacholine 10^{-4}M and were compared with paired t-tests. P values <0.05 (two-sided) were considered significant.

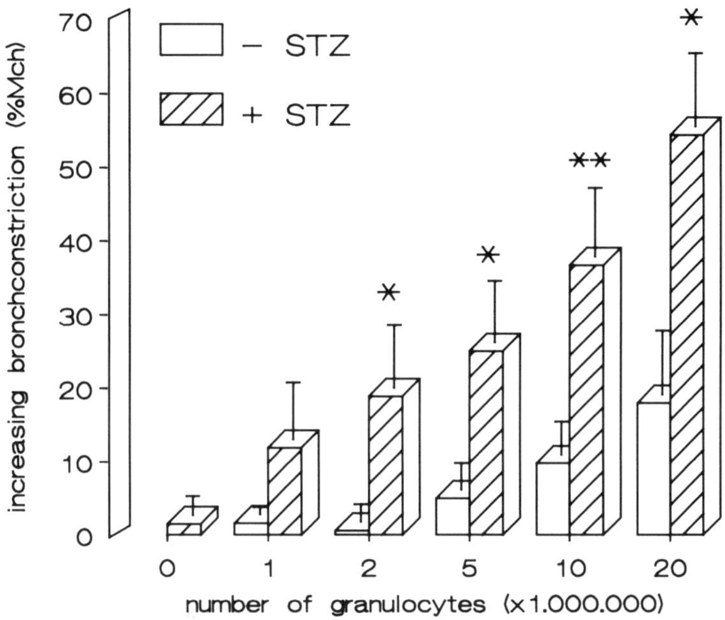

Figure 1. Response to increasing numbers of activated and un-activated granulocytes. * P<0.05, ** P<0.01 compared to response to unstimulated cells. n = 4-7.

RESULTS

STZ-activated granulocytes caused significantly more broncho-constriction than unstimulated granulocytes (Fig. 1). The magnitude of the contraction was proportional to the number of STZ-activated granulocytes present (P<0.001). NDGA and FPL 55712 both reduced the contraction to $10x10^6$ STZ-activated granulocytes by about 70% (P<0.001). Neither indomethacin nor mepyramine significantly changed the contractile effect of unactivated or activated granulocytes. The magnitude of the contraction to $10x10^6$ activated granulocytes correlated positively with the proportion of eosinophils among the granulocytes (P<0.01).

DISCUSSION

Our results show that incubation of isolated human airways with increasing numbers of STZ-activated granulocytes leads to increasing bronchoconstriction. Since STZ itself does not contract airway segments, the contraction to STZ-activated granulocytes must be secondary to activation of the granulocytes. This contraction is most likely due to the release of LTC_4/D_4 because it was reduced by about 70% both with NDGA and FPL 55712. The significant correlation between the number of activated eosinophils in the organ bath and the magnitude of the contraction suggests that eosinophils are implicated in the production of LTC_4 and that the role of neutrophils in the contraction is limited. Thus, our data support the possibility that activated eosinophils contribute to the LAR through the production of LTC_4.

Acknowledgements: The authors thank the Departments of Pathology, Pulmonology and Thoracic Surgery of the Ikazia and Leyenburg Hospitals, the Zuiderziekenhuis and the University Hospital of the Erasmus University for providing the lung tissue.
Supported by a grant of the Netherlands Asthma Foundation.

REFERENCES

Beasley, R., Roche, P.D., Roberts, J.A., and Holgate, S.T. (1989) Cellular events in the bronchi in mild asthma and after bronchial provocation. Am. Rev. Respir. Dis. 139, 806-817.

Booij-Noord, H., De Vries, K., Sluiter, H.J., and Orie, N.G.M. (1972) Late obstructive reaction to experimental inhalation of house dust extract. Clin. Allergy 1972 2, 43-61.

De Monchy, J.G.R., Kauffman, H.F., Venge, P., Koëter, G.H., Janssen, H.M., Sluiter, H.J., and De Vries K. (1985) Bronchoalveolar eosinophilia during allergen-induced late asthmatic reactions. Am. Rev. Respir. Dis. 131, 373-376.

Jongejan, R.C., De Jongste, J.C., Van Strik, R., Raatgeep, R.C., Bonta, I.L., and Kerrebijn, K.F. (1988) Measurement of human small airway smooth muscle function in vitro, comparison of bronchiolar strips and segments. J. Pharmacol. Meth. 20, 135-142.

Yazdanbakhsh, M., Eckmann, C.M., and Roos, D. (1985) Characterization of the interaction of human eosinophils and neutrophils with opsonized particles. J. Immunol. 135, 1378-1384.

PULMONARY SURFACTANT SECRETION IN THE TYPE II PNEUMOCYTES IN INFLAMED CONDITION

Y. Oda, H. Kai, K. Takaki, T. Yasunaga, K. Murahara, M. Kasano, K. Takahama and T. Miyata

Department of Pharmacological Science, Faculty of Pharmaceutical Science, Kumamoto University, 5-1, Oe-honmachi, Kumamoto, 862, Japan.

SUMMARY: Basal PC secretion in the type II pneumocytes from bronchitic rats was the same as that in the type II pneumocytes from normal rats. Neutrophils activated by opsonized zymosan or PMA, stimulated PC secretion in type II pneumocytes without causing any cell damage. The stimulation required close accession or attachment of neutrophils and type II pneumocytes and was not affected by the pretreatment with either SOD, catalase, AA861 or α_1-antitrypsin.

INTRODUCTION

The pulmonary surfactant, a phospholipid-rich material, is known to have some beneficial effects on pulmonary function or respiratory tract clearance. But the pathophysiological role of the pulmonary surfactant system remains unclear.

Previously, we have reported that pulmonary surfactant secretion was activated in bronchitic rats produced by long term sulfur dioxide exposure (Oda et al., 1989). To obtain some explanations for this phenomenon, two points have been investigated further with isolated and cultured type II pneumocytes in this study. First, basal PC secretion and pharmacological properties in type II pneumocytes were compared between normal rats and bronchitic rats produced by long term sulfur dioxide exposure. Second, we examined whether neutrophils, which were increased in broncho-alveolar lavage fluid of bronchitic rats, interact with type II pneumocytes.

MATERIALS AND METHODS

Bronchitic rats were produced by long term sulfur dioxide exposure as described previously (Oda et al., 1989).

Cell isolation and culture: Type II pneumocytes were isolated from adult male Wistar rats with or without bronchitis by tissue dissociation with trypsin and purified by incubation on petri-dish and on IgG-coated dish. The purity of the type II pneumocytes was 95%. The cells were suspended at 10^6 cells/ml in Dulbecco's modified Eagle Medium supplemented with 10% fetal bovine serum, ^{3}H-choline (2 µCi/ml), and antibiotics. The cells were cultured in a 5% CO_2/air atmosphere at 37°C for 18 hr. After 18 hr when the cell cultures established, pharmacological tests were done using the cells.

Neutrophils (PMNs) were isolated from atrial blood of normal rats by a common method. The PMNs were 90 to 95% pure as determined in Giemsa-stained smears.

PC secretion in type II pneumocytes from bronchitic rats: Type II pneumocytes from bronchitic rats were compared with that from normal rats on basal PC secretion and on activated secretion by 1-isoproterenol (10^{-5} M) and phorbol 12-myristate 13-acetate (PMA; 10^{-8} M).

PC secretion in type II pneumocytes in the presence of PMNs: PMNs (10^5 cells/ml) were added to the medium after cultivation of type II pneumocytes. After 5 min, opsonized zymosan (OPZ, 100 µg/ml) was added and ^{3}H-PC secretion in type II pneumocytes for 90 min was measured.

In some experiments, either superoxide dismutase (SOD, 2 units/ml), catalase (1000 units/ml), AA861 (10^{-4} M), or α_1-anti-trypsin (80 µg/ml) was added 10 min before PMNs activation.

After 90 min, the media and cells were removed and subjected to lipid extraction. The radioactivity in the total lipid fraction was routinely determined by a liquid scintillation counter. ^{3}H-PC secretion is expressed as percentage of radioactivity in a medium of total radioactivity deriving from medium and cells.

In cell-cell separation experiment, PMNs (10^5 cells/ml) and PMA (10 nM) were placed into plastic insert chambers separated approximately 2 mm from the type II pneumocytes by a 0.2 μ Millipore filter. The effect of PMNs was compared to positive control wells containing PMNs plus PMA without the separation chamber present.

Lactate dehydrogenase (LDH) amount as a marker of cytotoxicity was determined in all experiments by means of LDH kits (Nippon Shoji Co., Ltd.).

RESULTS

PC secretion in type II pneumocytes from bronchitic rats:
Basal PC secretion in the type II pneumocytes was not different between normal and bronchitic rats. The increasing responses in PC secretion by 1-isoproterenol and PMA slightly reduced in type II pneumocytes from bronchitic rats.

PC secretion in type II pneumocytes in the presence of PMNs:
The OPZ-activated PMNs caused an approximately 250% increase in the PC secretion comparing with control, whereas PMNs or OPZ alone showed no effect. The stimulation of PC secretion induced by activated PMNs was dependent on the number of PMNs (10^4 to 10^6 cells/ml). On the other hand, the release of LDH was not changed in the present study. The time course experiment indicated that the PC secretion was stimulated within 5 min and lasted for 10 min after PMNs activation.

The pretreatment with SOD, catalase, AA861, or α_1-antitrypsin had no effect on the stimulation of PC secretion by activated PMNs.

When PMNs were separated from type II pneumocytes by Millipore filters, the stimulatory action of activated PMNs was not produced.

DISCUSSION

Our results demonstrated that basal PC secretion in type II pneumocytes from bronchitic rats was not changed comparing with that in type II pneumocytes from normal rats. It seems, therefore, that the increase of pulmonary surfactant secretion in bronchitic rats is not due to the change of secretory function of the type II pneumocyte itself. However, the stimulatory action of 1-isoproterenol and PMA on PC secretion was reduced in type II pneumocytes from bronchitic rats, suggesting some changes caused on the plasma membrane in the type II pneumocytes, for example, the destruction of receptor.

It was presumed that inflammatory cells infiltrated on airway surface can be involved in the mechanism of the increased pulmonary surfactant secretion in bronchitic rats. So, the influence of PMNs coexistence with type II pneumocytes was investigated. Activated PMNs caused marked stimulation of PC secretion without giving cell damage.

It is known that activated PMNs release oxygen radicals, leukotrienes, and neutral proteases. However, the stimulation induced by activated PMNs was not reduced by the pretreatment with either of the inhibitors for these mediators, suggesting that these PMNs products are not primary factors in the stimulation of PC secretion. In addition, the stimulatory action required intimate contact between activated PMNs and type II pneumocytes.

The mechanism of the action induced by activated PMNs remains to be further investigated. Anyhow, PMNs infiltrated on airway surface may stimulate pulmonary surfactant secretion in the type II pneumocytes in inflammatory stage.

REFERENCES

Oda, Y., Isohama, Y., Kai, H., Okano, Y., Takahama, K., Miyata, T. (1989) Increased production and/or secretion of pulmonary surfactant in rats by long term sulfur dioxide exposure. J. Pharmacobio-Dyn. 12, 726-730.

SUPEROXIDE PRODUCTION BY BRONCHO-ALVEOLAR CELLS IS DIMINISHED IN PARAINFLUENZA-3 VIRUS TREATED GUINEA PIGS.

G. Folkerts, B. van Esch, M. Janssen en F.P. Nijkamp.

Dept. of Pharmacology, Faculty of Pharmacy, University of Utrecht, Catharijnesingel 60, 3511 GH Utrecht, The Netherlands.

SUMMARY: Guinea pig airways isolated 4, 8 and 16 days (but not 2 days) after intra-tracheal inoculation with parainfluenza-3 virus *In Vivo* respond hyperreactive to contractile stimuli.
In the present study it is shown that the virus-induced airway hyperresponsiveness is associated with a decreased Superoxide production by broncho-alveolar cells after additional stimulation with parainfluenza-3 virus.

INTRODUCTION

Virus-induced bronchial hyperreactivity may be important, not only as a clinical entity, but also as a "model" to study basic mechanisms in the pathogenesis of asthma (Busse, 1990). Efforts have been made to study virus-induced asthma, and many have focused on mediator release by inflammatory cells. To study more in detail this issue we infected guinea pig airways by intra-tracheal inoculation of parainfluenza-3 (PI-3). This results in a significantly enhanced airway response to contractile stimuli *In Vitro* 4, 8 and 16 days (but not 2 days) after virus treatment (Folkerts & Nijkamp, 1990).
The aim of the present study was to investigate whether broncho-alveolar cells (BAC) can be stimulated by PI-3 virus *In Vitro*, by measurement of Superoxide (SO) production. A second objective was to study whether the PI-3 induced SO-production of the BAC was changed 2, 4, 8 and 16 days after the guinea pigs had been inoculated with the virus *In Vivo*.

MATERIALS AND METHODS

Specified pathogen free male Dunkin Hartley guinea pigs (400-500) were housed under controlled conditions in an isolator. The virus suspension (TCID50 = $10^{8.9}$/ml) was centrifugated at 100.000 g and resuspended in; a) 10 times less volume saline for inoculation, b) in 2 times less volume Krebs-buffer for stimulation of BAC. Growth medium was treated in the same way. The animals received 0.1 ml saline or PI-3 intra-tracheally under a light ether anaesthesia. Guinea pigs were killed with pentobarbitone sodium (30 mg $100g^{-1}$ body weight) intra-peritoneally, 2, 4, 8, and 16 days after inoculation. BAC were obtained by lavage of the lungs as described previously (Folkerts et al., 1988). The recovered cells were washed and brought to a concentration of 5 x 10^6cells/ml. Generation of SO was assayed by measuring the reduction of ferricytochrome c (Horse heart type VI, Sigma Chemical Co., St. Louis, MO) by using a modification of the method described by Babior et al., (1973). The standard reaction mixture contained 1 x 10^6BAC, 90mM ferricytochrome c with or without 200ul virus suspension. Krebs-bicarbonate buffer was added to make a final volume of 1 ml. Paired reaction mixtures with and without Superoxide dismutase (E.C. 1.15.1.1, Bovine blood type I, Sigma; 100 ug/reaction mixture) were employed. Nanomoles of reduced ferricytochrome c were determined from the increase in absorbance at 550nm by using the molar extinction coefficient $E_{550}=2.1x10^4M^{-1}cm^{-1}$. Changes in SO-production between groups were tested with Student's unpaired t test.

RESULTS

Two days after saline inoculation the SO-production by BAC stimulated *In Vitro* with PI-3 was 80% enhanced (from 6.5 ± 1.0 to 11.7 ± 1.7 nmole/10^6BAC/15min, $P<0.05$) above basal values. This stimulation was the same in BAC obtained from guinea pigs 2 days after PI-3 infection (93 %, from 6.1 ± 0.6 to 11.8 ± 1.7 nmole).

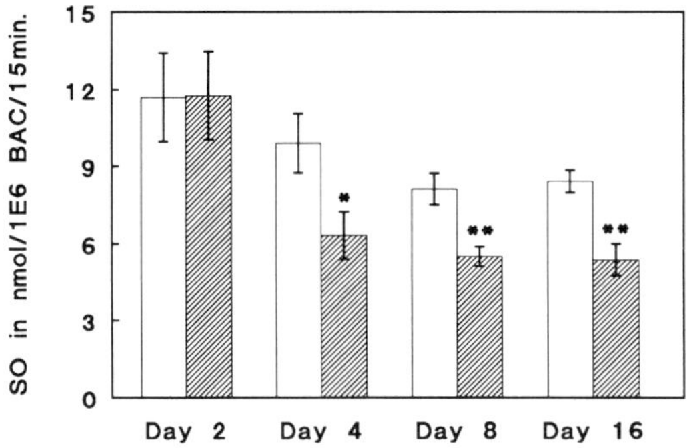

Figure, PI-3 virus induced Superoxide production by BAC obtained 2, 4, 8, and 16 days after the guinea pigs were inoculated with saline or PI-3 virus. N=6-12, *$P<0.05$, **$P<0.01$.

In contrast, the virus-induced SO-production of BAC obtained from animals 4, 8 and 16 days after PI-3 inoculation was significantly decreased (36, 32 and 36 % respectively) as compared with the control groups (Figure).

DISCUSSION

In the present study it is shown that BAC can be stimulated by PI-3 virus as was demonstrated by an increase in SO-production. In addition it was demonstrated that 4, 8 and 16 days (but not 2 days) after virus inoculation *In Vivo*, the BAC responded less to additional PI-3 stimulation *In Vitro*. Interestingly, on the day were no difference in SO-production was observed (day 2), also no difference in airway reactivity to contractile stimuli *In Vitro* occured (Folkerts & Nijkamp, 1990). Further, on the days were SO-production by BAC was decreased, hyperreactivity of the respiratory airways was detected (Folkerts & Nijkamp, 1990). Therefore, a relationship between changes in SO-production by BAC and changes in responsiveness of the airways seems to be present.

The inoculated viruses in the guinea pig airways In Vivo will be eliminated by BAC. During phagocytosis of PI-3, SO is generated in the lung. BAC will probably become exhausted and/or the neuraminidase receptors will become occupied, and this can explain why those cells generate less SO after additional stimulation with PI-3 virus *In Vitro*.

Free oxygen radicals mediate a number of (patho-)physiological processes (Nijkamp & Henricks, 1988). For instance they stimulate the liberation of mediators from mast cells (Mannaioni & Masini, 1988), which in turn can influence airway responsiveness (Weiss & Bellino, 1986). In addition, free radicals can directly act on cell membrane lipids/proteins and subsequently modulate reactivity of airways (Nijkamp & Henricks, 1988).

In conclusion, PI-3 virus can stimulate BAC to generate reactive oxygen radicals, which in turn may modulate directly or indirectly respiratory airway reactivity.

REFERENCES

Busse, W.W. (1990) Respiratory infections: Their role in airway responsiveness and the pathogenesis of asthma. J. All. Clin, Immunol. 85, 671-683.

Folkerts, G., and Nijkamp, F.P. (1990) Does stimulation of broncho-alveolar cells by viruses lead to respiratory airway hyperreactivity in the guinea pig. Eur. J. Pharmacol. 183, 188-189.

Folkerts, G., Henricks, P.A.J., Slootweg, P.J., and Nijkamp, F.P. (1988) Endotoxin-induced inflammation and injury of the guinea pig respiratory airways cause bronchial hyporeactivity. Am. Rev. Resp. Dis. 137, 1441-1448.

Babior, B.M., Kipnes, R.S., and Curnutte, J.T. (1973) Biological defence mechanisms. The production by leukocytes of Superoxide a potential bactericidal agent. J. Clin. Invest. 52, 741-744.

Nijkamp, F.P., and Henricks P.A.J. (1988) Free radicals in pulmonary disease. In: Asthma: Basic mechanisms and clinical management (Barnes, P.J., Rodger, I.W., and N.C. Thomson, Eds), Academic Press Limited, London, pp. 315-323.

Mannaioni, P.F., and Masini, E. (1988) The release of histamine by free radicals. Free Radical Biol. Med. 5, 177-197.

Weiss, E.B., and Bellino, J.R. (1986) Leukotriene-associated toxic oxygen metabolites induce airway hyperreactivity. Chest 89 (5), 709-716.

AAS 31:
Mediators in
Airway Hyperreactivity

OXIDATIVE STRESS AND RECEPTOR RESPONSES IN GUINEA-PIG TRACHEAL TISSUE

Cees J.A. Doelman, Janneke F. de Vlieger, R. Corinne Sprong and Aalt Bast

Department of Pharmacochemistry, Faculty of Chemistry, Vrije Universiteit, De Boelelaan 1083, 1081 HV Amsterdam, The Netherlands.

SUMMARY: Reactive oxygen species are formed during inflammatory reactions in the lung. Alveolar macrophages and neutrophils and eosinophils produce superoxide anions, hydrogen peroxide, hydroxyl radicals and singlet oxygen. Neutrophils and eosinophils produce also hypochlorous acid. We now present the effects of hydrogen peroxide and hypochlorous acid on muscarinic and beta-adrenergic receptor responses of guinea pig tracheal tissue. Hydrogen peroxide (up to 10 mM) has no effect on these receptor responses, but in contrast hypochlorous acid destructs the muscarinic and beta-adrenergic receptor response. The beta-adrenergic receptor response is more susceptible to hypochlorous acid treatment than the muscarinic receptor response. This indicates that hypochlorous acid induces an autonomic imbalance between parasympatic and sympatic receptor responses in the guinea pig trachea.

Reactive oxygen species seem to play a role in the genesis of several lung pathological conditions like the adult respiratory distress syndrome, emphysema, pulmonary inflammation (asthma), coalmine workers pneumoconiosis (Heffner and Repine, 1989; Doelman et al., 1990). Stimulated macrophages, monocytes, neutrophils and eosinophils produce superoxide anions by the membrane-bound enzyme NADPH oxidase. Superoxide anions dismutate to hydrogen peroxide either enzymatically (superoxide dismutase) or non-enzymatically. In the presence of iron, superoxide anions and hydrogen peroxide together produce hydroxyl radicals. Myeloperoxidase (released by stimulated neutrophils) and eosinophil peroxidase (released by eosinophils) convert hydrogen peroxide to hypochlorous acid (Southorn and Powis, 1988). Reactive oxygen species (ROS) are able to destruct DNA or RNA, inactivate proteins and induce a stepwise deterioration of lipid structures (named lipid peroxidation). During lipid peroxidation toxic aldehydes, such as 4-hydroxy-2,3-transnonenal (4-HNE) are formed (Vaca et al., 1988)

ROS seem to play a role in the genesis of bronchial hyperreactivity. Meltzer et al. (1989) and Postma et al. (1988) found a correlation between the measured bronchial hyperreactivity in asthmatics and patients with chronic obstructive pulmonary diseases (COPD) and the amount of superoxide anions produced by their blood leukocytes. Moreover Weiss and Bellino (1986 a,b) observed that hyperreactivity induced by leukotriene D_4 or anaphylaxis in guinea pigs tracheal tissue *in vitro* is inhibited by the addition of superoxide dismutase. This indicates that superoxide anions induce hyperreactivity of the guinea pig pulmonary smooth muscle.

In order to determine the role of ROS in the genesis of bronchial hyperreactivity, we investigated the effects of hydrogen peroxide and hypochlorous acid on the muscarinic and beta-adrenergic receptor responses of the guinea pig tracheal smooth muscle.

MATERIALS AND METHODS

Male guinea pigs (350-450 g) were killed by cervical dislocation and the trachea was rapidly excised and mounted in a Krebs buffer solution (Doelman et al., 1988). Small transverse strips, containing 1 cartilage ring were cut form the trachea and mounted in an organ bath containing Krebs buffer solution at 37° continuously gassed with a mixture of 95% O_2 and 5% CO_2 in order to maintain oxygen tension and a pH of 7.4. Either methacholine or (-)-isoprenaline dose response curves were recorded and between each dose response curves a washing period of 35 min. (with 7 intermediate changes of buffer solution) was applied in order to remove all used drugs. After 3 dose reponse curves, the tracheal strips were incubated for 30 min. with either hydrogen peroxide or hypochlorous acid and after a washing period of 35 min. a dose response curve was recorded.

RESULTS

Incubation of guinea pig tracheal tissue with hydrogen peroxide (concentrations up to 10 mM) did not affect the methacholine dose response curve (-log EC_{50} of 6.12 ± 0.04). Also the (-)-isoprenaline dose response curve of the guinea pig trachea was not changed after hydrogen peroxide pretreatment (up to 10 mM).

In contrast, after 1 mM hypochlorous acid pretreatment for 30 min, the -logEC_{50} for methacholine was decreased from 6.12 ± 0.04 to 5.93 ± 0.05 and also the maximal effect of methacholine was diminished from 114 ± 2 % to 74 ± 7 %. Incubation with 10 mM hypochlorous acid resulted in a -log EC_{50} for methacholine of 5.56 ± 0.02 and a maximal effect of 21 ± 2 %.

The β-adrenergic receptor response was also affected by hypochlorous acid pretreatment. Incubation with 0.1 mM hypochlorous acid resulted in a slight decrease of -log EC_{50} for (-)-isoprenaline form 9.06 ± 0.04 (control) to 8.91 ± 0.09. No change was observed of the maximal effect. Incubation with 1 mM hypochlorous acid resulted in a -log EC_{50} of 8.50 ± 0.10. After pretreatment with a concentration of 10 mM hypochlorous acid, (-)-isoprenaline did not induce any relaxation.

DISCUSSION

In contrast to rat tracheal tissue (Doelman et al., 1988), hydrogen peroxide did not affect the muscarinic and β-adrenergic receptor response of guinea-pig tracheal smooth muscle. These results are in accordance to the effects obtained by Rhoden and Barnes (1989). Hypochlorous acid, which can be produced by stimulated neutrophils and eosinophils, destructs dose dependently the muscarinic and β-adrenergic receptor response of guinea-pig tracheal smooth muscle. When the guinea-pig tracheal smooth muscle is incubated with 10 mM HOCl, still methacholine contracts the smooth muscle, but addition of (-)-isoprenaline to the smooth muscle did not induce relaxation. This indicates that the β-adrenergic receptor response of the guinea pig trachea is more susceptible to HOCl treatment than the muscarinic receptor response. We thus conclude that hypochlorous acid can cause an autonomic imbalance between sympatic and parasympatic receptor responses.

Asthmatic lungs are hyperresponsive to contractile stimuli and hyporesponsive to relaxing stimuli like (-)-isoprenaline (Lemanske and Kaliner, 1990). Incubation with hypochlorous acid causes also an autonomic imbalance between parasympatic and sympatic receptor responses. We conclude that hypochlous acid may contribute to the genesis of bronchial hyperresponsiveness.

Acknowledgement: This study was financially supported by the Dutch Asthma Foundation (grant nr. 87-30).

REFERENCES:

Doelman, C.J.A.; Kramer, K., Timmerman, H., Bast, A. (1988) Vitamin E and selenium regulate the balance between beta-adrenergic and muscarinic responses in rat lungs. FEBS Lett. 233: 427-431.

Doelman, C.J.A.; Leurs, R.; Oosterom, W.C.; Bast, A. (1990) Mineral dust exposure and free radical mediated lung damage. Exp. Lung Res. 16: 41-55.

Heffner, J.E.; Repine, J.E. (1989) Pulmonary strategies of antioxidant defense. State of the art. Am. Rev. Respir. Dis. 140: 531-554.

Lemanske, R.F., Kaliner, M.A. (1990) Autonomic nervous system abnormalities and asthma. Am. Rev. Respir. Dis. 141: S157-S161.

Postma, D.S., Renkema, T.E.J., Noordhoek, J.A., Faber, H., Sluiter, H.J., Kauffman, H. (1998) Association between nonspecific bronchial hyperreactivity and superoxide anion production by polymorphonuclear leukocytes in chronic airflow obstruction. Am. Rev. Respir. Dis. 137: 57-61.

Rhoden, K.J., Barnes, P.J. (1989) Effect of hydrogen peroxide on guinea-pig tracheal smooth muscle in vitro: role of cyclo-oxygenase and airway epithelium. Br. J. Pharmacol. 98: 325-330.

Southorn, P.A.; Powis, G. (1988) Free radicals in medicine. I. Chemical nature and biological reactions. Mayo Clin. Proc. 63: 3881-389.

Vaca, C.E.; Wilhelm, J.; Harms-Ringdahl, M. (1988) Interaction of lipid peroxidation products with DNA. A review. Mutation Res. 195: 137-149.

Weiss, E.B., Bellino, J.R. (1986 a) Superoxide anion generation during airway anaphylaxis. Int Arch. Allergy Appl. Immunol. 80: 211-213.

Weiss, E.B., Bellino, J.R. (1986 b) Leukotriene-associated toxic oxygen metabolites induces airway hyperreactivity. Chest 89: 709-716.

AAS 31:
Mediators in
Airway Hyperreactivity

CYTOKINES AND BRONCHIAL HYPERREACTIVITY

Rafeul Alam

Allergy Division, Department of Medicine, The University of Texas, Medical Branch, Galveston, TX 77550, USA

SUMMARY: Cytokines and interleukins are a potent group of molecules that is primarily involved in maintaining homeostasis. These molecules regulate the growth and function of many cells of the immune system including eosinophils, mast cells/basophils and others. Activation of the later cells by cytokines may play a crucial role in the development of allergic inflammation of the airways. The importance of cytokines in the pathogenesis of bronchial hyperreactivity and asthma has been reviewed in this paper.

One of the cardinal features of asthma is bronchial hyperreactivity. The cause of bronchial hyperreactivity is multiple, and the pathophysiologic basis is complex. There exist a number of hypotheses that tend to explain the pathogenesis of bronchial hyperreactivity. They include:

1. autonomic nervous dysfunction:
   - a: heightened excitatory response:
     - 1). increased cholinergic response, and
     - 2). enhanced non-adrenergic non-cholinergic response;
   - b: impaired inhibitory (dilatory) response:
     - 1). decreased adrenergic response, and
     - 2). reduced non-adrenergic non-cholinergic inhibitory response;
   - c: abnormal neuropeptide release at the sensory nerve endings.
2. chronic inflammation characterized by:

a: increased eosinophils, metachromatic cells and others,

b: augmented mediator release from inflammatory cells.

3. desquamation of airway epithelium and loss of epithelial relaxing effect.
4. heightened airway mucosal permeability.

These hypotheses are not mutually exclusive, and in fact, they are complementary to one another. Chronic inflammation following an airway allergic reaction can initiate a sequence of events that can lead to all of the above mentioned phenomena.

The presence of increased amounts of inflammatory mediators such as histamine (1), tryptase (2), MBP, and ECP (3) and cells such as eosinophils and metachromatic cells (4) have been a consistent finding in the bronchoalveolar lavage fluids and bronchial mucosa in patients with asthma. MBP (5) and tryptase (6) can cause bronchial hyperreactivity. The mechanism of cellular infiltration and mediator release have been the subject of extensive research in recent years. One group of molecules that play a key role in the induction of inflammation is integrins. Wegner et al (7) have used antibody against one member of the integrin family, namely intercellular adhesion molecule-1 (ICAM-1). They have shown that pretreatment with anti-ICAM-1 antibody abrogates pulmonary eosinophilia and reverses bronchial hyperreactivity in the experimental model of asthma in monkeys. In addition to integrins, attention has been focused on the role played by a multitude of cytokines and interleukins that have been identified recently.

CYTOKINES AND EOSINOPHILS

One of the characteristic features of allergic diseases is eosinophilia. There exists compelling evidence that eosinophils play a major role in the pathogenesis of chronic allergic inflammation and bronchial hyperreactivity. These cells are the major source of spasmogenic LTC_4 and LTD_4. The granule content of these cells including MBP, ECP, EDN/RNAse are cytotoxic to many cells, and cause excessive tissue damage and desquamation of the respiratory epithelium in asthmatic patients. IL-5 is an eosinophil growth factor, and stimulates bone marrow stem cells to differentiate into eosinophils (8). IL-5 appears to regulate eosinophilia. The administration of anti-IL-5 antibody to mice prior to parasitic infestation inhibits peripheral blood and tissue eosinophilia (9). IL-3 also stimulates eosinophil growth and makes them hypodense (10). Recently, GM-CSF has been identified as another cytokine that prime eosinophils for enhanced LTC_4 synthesis (11). These results, suggest that cytokines may play a pivotal role in upregulating eosinophilic inflammation in the airways and contribute to the development of bronchial hyperreactivity.

CYTOKINES AND IgE ANTIBODY SYNTHESIS

IgE-mediated allergic reaction represents the initial event in the pathogenesis of allergic asthma. The synthesis of IgE is strictly regulated by an interplay of a number of cytokines including IL-4, CD23, IL-6 and gamma-interferon (12). IL-4 stimulates precursor B cells for clonal expansion and differentiation. This interleukin also induces the expression of CD23 on activated B cells, and causes the release soluble CD23 (a low molecular weight B cell growth factor). Subsequent action of IL-4 and CD23 in combination induces preferential synthesis of IgE antibody. Pretreatment of mice with anti-IL-4 antibody abrogates parasite-induced IgE response (13). Another T cell product, interferon-gamma antagonizes the action of IL-4 and inhibits IgE synthesis.

CYTOKINES AND THE GROWTH OF MAST CELLS/BASOPHILS

The intricate relationship between T cells and the growth and differentiation of mast cells has been investigated and recognized in the 60's and 70's. It is now well established that IL-3, a pluripotential stem cell growth factor, is instrumental in the growth and differentiation of mast cells and basophils from stem cell precursors (for review see ref. 14). IL-4 exerts an additive effect on mast cell growth. The ultimate phenotypic differentiation (connective vs mucosal mast cells) is determined by as yet unidentified local cytokines produced in the milieu of mucosa and connective tissue. In the later instance, fibroblasts have been shown to modulate the differentiation of connective tissue mast cells. IL-3 also induces de novo synthesis of histidine decarboxylase, an enzyme that catalyzes the production of histamine.

MAST CELLS AND THE SYNTHESIS OF CYTOKINES

Mast cells synthesize a multitude of inflammatory mediators that are released immediately upon activation. Recent studies have shown that mast cells also produce a number of cytokines including IL-3, -4, -5 and -6, GM-CSF and TNF (15-17). The synthesis and release of these cytokines take place 6 hr after activation, temporally coinciding with the late phase reaction. The production of cytokines points to a hitherto unrecognized mechanism of chronic inflammation sustained by mast cells.

CYTOKINES AND MAST CELLS/BASOPHILS

The involvement of mast cells and basophils have been recognized in many pathologic conditions where IgE antibody appears to be absent. This observation led to the emergence of the concept that mast cell/basophil activation may occur via cytokines (Table I).

Table I. Activity of different cytokines on basophil mediator release.

Release	Enhancement	Inhibition	No Effect
IL-3	IL-3	IL-8-beta	IL-4, -5, -6
GM-CSF	GM-CSF	HRIF	TNF
CTAP III	IL-1		TGF-beta
NAP-2	IL-2		PDGF-BB
HRF			Endothelin
			Beta-thromboglobulin

Thueson et al (18) first demonstrated that mononuclear cell culture supernatant releases histamine from basophils, and that the active substance is distinct from IgE antibody or C5a. Subsequent studies from a number of laboratories confirmed this observation (19-22). Histamine releasing factors (HRF) represent a heterogeneous group of substances that release histamine and leukotrienes from mast cells and basophils. HRF is produced by many cells including T cells, B cells, monocytes, neutrophils and platelets (21-23).

We have investigated the identity of HRF with other cytokines. IL-3 appears to be the most active molecule amongst cytokines, although it releases histamine from basophils of select allergic donors only (24-26). In contrast, mononuclear cell-derived HRF releases histamine from basophils obtained from allergic as well as normal non-allergic donors. In addition, the activity of mononuclear cell-derived HRF is not blocked by anti-IL-3 antibody (25). GM-CSF is another cytokine that releases small amounts of histamine from some select donors (24, 25). There are reports of histamine release by IL-1 (27) and IL-8 (28), but the results are disputed by others (29, 30). In addition to its direct histamine releasing effect, IL-3 primes basophils for degranulation by other agents. Preincubation of basophils with IL-3 causes enhanced histamine release to anti-IgE and C5a (31, 32). These observations suggest that IL-3 plays a key role in the development as well as function of mast cells and basophils.

As stated earlier, mononuclear cell-HRF appears distinct from most other cytokines. Several species of HRF have been purified by Baeza et al (33) and by us (34). Partial amino acid sequence of one species of HRF (10-12 KD) is known thus far (35). This species appears to be identical to connective tissue activating protein III (CTAP III) and its cleavage product, neutrophil activating peptide-2 (NAP-2). CTAP III is produced by platelets, and CTAP I is secreted by lymphocytes. CTAP III stimulates the synthesis of collagen and glycosaminoglycan by fibroblasts (36). The purification of some more potent, and perhaps novel HRF is anticipated in the near future.

HRF, BRONCHIAL HYPERREACTIVITY AND ASTHMA

The involvement of HRF in asthma has been the subject of a number of investigations. The following observations suggest that HRF may play an important role in the pathogenesis of asthma.

<u>a. Heightened production of HRF in allergic asthma.</u>

Mononuclear cells (MNC) from asthmatic patients spontaneously produce relatively high amounts of HRF (19, 37). This production is enhanced upon incubation of MNC with specific allergens (37). The magnitude of spontaneous production of HRF highly correlates ($r = -0.86$; $P<0.01$) with the severity of asthma as assessed by symptom score (Fig. 1) and bronchial hyperreactivity (PC_{20} for histamine) in asthmatic patients (38). Spontaneous HRF production increases during the natural exposure to the allergens in the pollen season and this increased production is correlated with the symptom score of the patients (39).

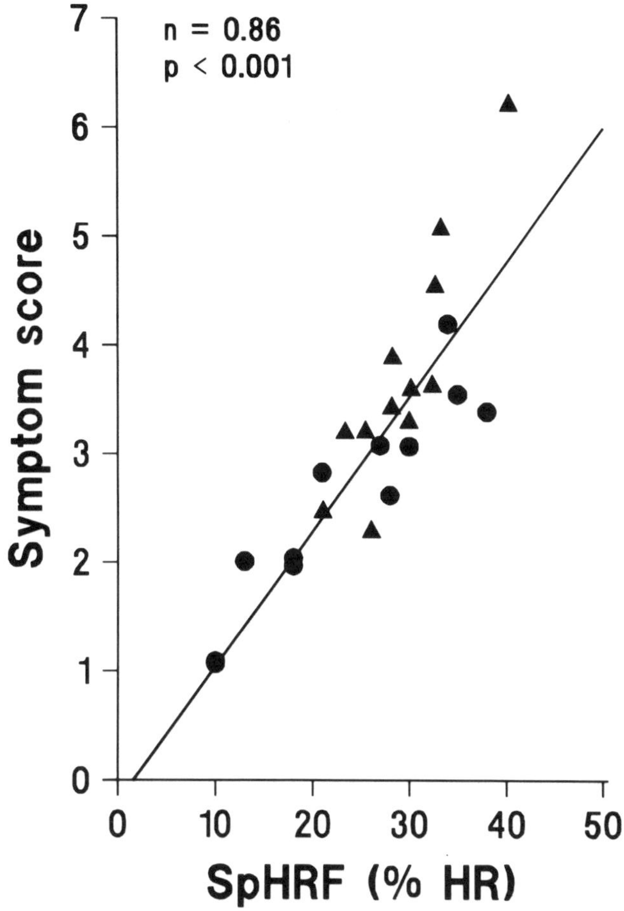

Fig. 1. The correlation between spontaneous HRF synthesis by MNC from allergic asthmatic patients and their symptom score. Symptom scores during the grass pollen season were obtained from twenty four asthmatic patients with grass allergy. MNC from the patients were isolated and cultured in the middle of pollen season. Supernatants were assayed for histamine releasing activity using basophils from a single healthy donor. (Reproduced with permission, Kuna et al, J. Allergy Clin. Immunol. 1989, 83, 816).

b. Association of HRF with late phase allergic reactions.

Kuna et al have recently demonstrated that the synthesis of HRF by MNC increases significantly after allergen inhalation challenge only in patients who develop a late phase asthmatic reaction (40). Patients with an immediate asthmatic reaction did not show increased HRF synthesis. The increase in HRF synthesis occurred at 6 hr and it tended to correlate with the fall in FEV_1 in the late phase reaction. In agreement with this study, Warner et al have previously detected an HRF-like activity in skin blister fluids obtained from late but not immediate allergic reactions (41). Since mast cell/basophil mediators are released in the late phase allergic reactions, it is possible that HRF may be the cause of basophil/mast cell activation in the late phase reaction.

c. Reduction of HRF after immunotherapy

If HRF is involved in the pathogenesis of asthma, specific immunotherapy should reduce the synthesis of HRF. This hypothesis was tested by Kuna et al in a double-blind placebo-controlled randomized study with 24 patients (39). Immunotherapy initially abrogated the seasonal rise in the production of HRF and then significantly reduced the production in the clinically benefitted patients. Immunotherapy also decreased the allergen-induced HRF production by MNC in vitro (Fig. 2). In an uncontrolled study, Hsieh et al have recently confirmed these observations (42).

d. Increased sensitivity of basophils from allergic patients to HRF.

Although basophils from most donors respond to HRF, cells from allergic and/or asthmatic patients are more sensitive to HRF than cells from healthy controls (43, 44). This provides HRF a unique capability to interact with basophils infiltrating the target tissue in the late phase reaction in allergic subjects.

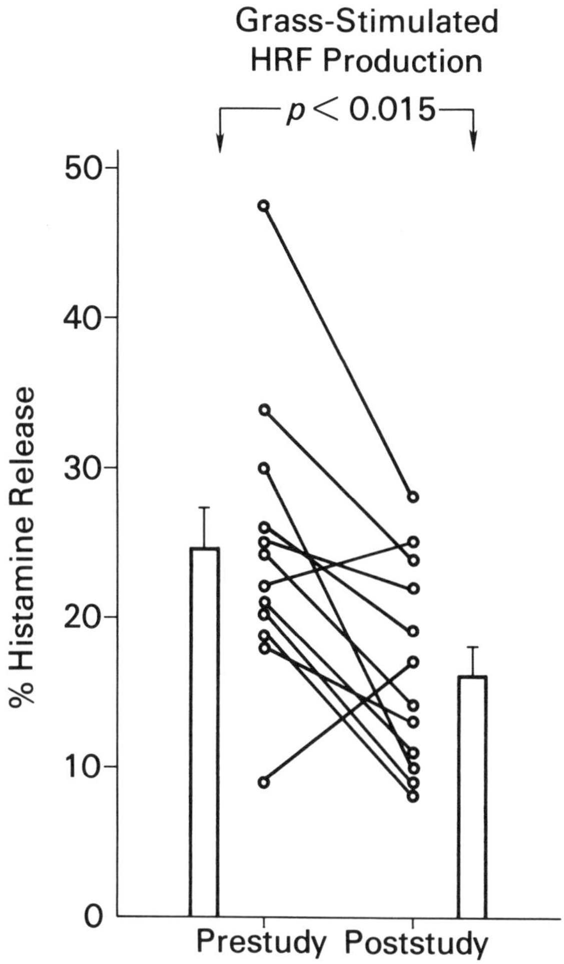

Fig. 2. Effect of two years of immunotherapy on grass-stimulated HRF synthesis by MNC. Twelve asthmatic patients received preseasonal immunotherapy for two consecutive years. MNC from the patients were cultured in the presence of grass allergens, and the supernatants were assayed for HRF activity using basophils from a single donor. The grass-stimulated HRF synthesis by MNC from these patients before and after two years of immunotherapy are shown. (Reproduced with permission, Kuna et al. J. Allergy Clin. Immunol. 1989, 83, 816).

e. IgE-dependency of some species of HRF.

As noted earlier, basophils from allergic patients respond better to HRF. The mechanism of this heightened response has been investigated by MacDonald et al (43) and by us (44). It has been shown that the removal of IgE from the surface of basophils abolishes the response to HRF. The response to HRF can be restored by incubating the basophils with serum or IgE from some allergic patients but not normal subjects or myeloma IgE. On the basis of these observations, MacDonald et al (43) and Lichtenstein et al (45) have postulated the existence of a distinct type of IgE, so-called IgE+ that render basophils responsive to HRF. Further studies by MacDonald et al (43) have established that one single species mononuclear cell-derived HRF is IgE-dependent and others not. IgE+ represents a special form of glycosylated IgE. The addition of inhibitors of glycosylation to B cell cultures blocks the synthesis of IgE+. These studies pointed to a novel role of IgE.

f. Intrinsic asthma

Although much is known about etiologic factors and mechanism of allergic asthma, the pathogenesis of intrinsic asthma remains a major challenge to date. Since HRF represents a novel mechanism of mediator release, it is tempting to speculate that this mechanism is involved in intrinsic asthma. We have reported that MNC from intrinsic asthmatic patients spontaneously produce high amounts of HRF (46). The production is stimulated by culture of MNC with bacterial antigens in some patients (47). Since infectious agents have been implicated in the pathogenesis of this form of asthma, it is possible that the stimulation of HRF production by these and other unidentified agents contributes to the development of intrinsic asthma.

The exact role played by cytokines in asthma remains to be elucidated in the future. We speculate that the high spontaneous HRF production provides a mechanism of continued mediator release in the target organ and leads to the development of bronchial hyperreactivity and chronic asthma.

HISTAMINE RELEASE INHIBITORY FACTOR (HRIF)

We have described another group of cytokines that inhibit HRF-induced histamine release from basophils (48). At least three species of HRIF in the MW range of 8-10 KD, 15-25 KD and 40-45 KD have been identified by gel filtration, anion exchange and reverse phase HPLC. HRIF inhibits HRF-induced histamine release from basophils. It does not affect histamine release by anti-IgE, C5a and FMLP. We have recently established that IL-8-beta (77 amino acid peptide) also inhibits HRF-induced histamine release from basophils.

Like HRIF, IL-8 is specifically antagonizes HRF and does not affect histamine release by anti-IgE, C5a and FMLP. On reverse phase HPLC, both IL-8 and purified 8 KD HRIF have identical retention time. The establishment of actual relationship of 8 KD HRIF to IL-8-beta will require sequence analysis. IL-8-gamma (72 amino acid peptide) is a potent neutrophil chemotactic/ activating factor (49). Interestingly Gimbrone et al demonstrated that IL-8-beta inhibits adhesion of neutrophils to endothelium implying an anti-chemotactic activity (50). The mechanism of this agonistic-antagonistic property of two structurally similar molecules is unknown. Nonetheless, it appears that cytokines may not only cause inflammation, but also act as antiiflammatory agents under specific conditions which is perhaps important in restoring homeostasis.

We have detected the activity of both HRIF and HRF in the BAL fluid obtained from healthy subjects (51). The presence of HRIF was in abundance since it was detectable in the unconcentrated BAL. HRF activity was measurable only in highly concentrated (10-50x) BAL fluid. These results suggest that HRIF may play a physiologic role in the downregulation of mediator release in the airways.

It is apparent from this brief review that the cytokine network encompasses a broad range of potent effector molecules capable of mounting immunologic response in the form of both immediate and late allergic reactions as well as chronic inflammation. The importance of cytokines and interleukins lies in the fact that many of them are secreted in the early phase of immunologic response. The implication is that by interfering with the function of these effector molecules one may be able to safeguard excessive host damage and prevent diseases like bronchial asthma.

REFERENCES

1. Casale, T.B., Wood, D., Richerson, H.B., Trapp, S., Metzger, W.J., Zaval, D., and Hunninghake, G.W. (1987). Elevated bronchoalveolar lavage fluid histamine levels in allergic asthmatics are associated with methacholine bronchial hyperresponsiveness. J. Clin. Invest. 79, 1197-1203.
2. Wenzel, S.E., Fowler III, A.A., and Schwartz, L.B. (1988). Activation of pulmonary mast cells by bronchoalveolar allergen challenge. In vivo release of histamine and tryptase in atopic subjects with and without asthma. Am. Rev. Respir. Dis. 137, 1002-1008.
3. Frigas, E., and Gleich, G.J. (1986). The eosinophil and the pathophysiology of asthma. J. Allergy Clin. Immunol. 77, 527-537.
4. Wardlaw, A.J., Dunnette, S., Gleich, G.J., Collins, and Kay, A.B. (1988). Eosinophils and mast cells in bronchoalveolar lavage in subjects with mild asthma. Relationship to bronchial hyperreactivity. Am. Rev. Respir. Dis. 137, 62-69.
5. Flavahan, N.A., Slifman, N.R., Gleich, G.J., and Vanhoutte, P.M. (1988). Human eosinophil major basic protein causes hyperreactivity of respiratoiy smooth muscle. Am. Rev. Respir. Dis. 138, 685-688.
6. Sekizawa, K., Caughey, G. J., Lazarus, S., Gold, W.M., and Nadel, J.A. (1989). Mast cell tryptase causes airway smooth muscle hyperreponsiveriess in dogs. J. Clin. Invest. 83, 175-179.
7. Wegner, C.D., Gundel, R.H., Reilly, P., Haynes, N., Letts, G., and Rothlein, R. (1990). Intercellular adhesion molecule-

1 (ICAM-1) in the pathogenesis of asthma. Science 247, 456-459.
8. Clutterbuck, E., Shields, J.G, Gordon, J., Smith, S.H., Boyd, A., Callard, R.E., Campbell, H.D., Young, I.G., and Sanderson, C.J. (1987). Recombinant human interleukin 5 is an eosinophil differentiation factor but has no activity in standard B cell growth factor assay. Eur. J. Immunol. 17, 1743-1750.
9. Coffman, R.L., Seymour, B.W.P., Hudak, S., Jackson, J., and Rennick, D. (1989). Antibody to interleukin-5 inhibits helminth-induced eosinophilia in mice. Science 245, 308-310.
10. Rothenberg, M.E., Owen, Jr, W.F., Siverstein, D.S., Woods, J., Soberman, R.J., Austen, K.F., and Stevens, R.L. (1988). Human eosinophils have prolonged survival, enhance functional properties, and become hypodense when exposed to human interleukin 3. J. Clin. Invest. 81, 1986-1992.
11. Howell, C.J., Pujol, J-L., Crea, A.E.G., Davidson, R., Gearing, A.J.H., Godard, Ph., and Lee, T. (1989). Identification of an alveolar macrophage-derived activity in bronchial asthma that enhances leukotriene C_4 generation by human eosinophils stimulated by ionophore A23187 as a granulocyte-macrophage colony-stimulating factor. Am. Rev. Respir. Dis. 140, 1340-1347.
12. Snapper, C.M., and Paul, W.E. (1987). Interferon-gamma and B cell stimulatory factor-1 reciprocally regulate Ig isotype production. Science 236, 944-947.
13. Finkelman, F.D., Katon, I.M., Urban, Jr., J.F., Snaffer, C.M., Ohara, J., and Paul, W.E. (1986). Suppression of in vivo polyclonal IgE responses by monoclonal antibody to the lymphokine B cell stimulatory factor 1. Proc. Natl. Acad. Sci. U.S.A. 83, 9675-9678.
14. Stevens, R.L., and Austen, K.F. (1989). Recent advances in the cellular and molecular biology of mast cells. Immunol. Today 10, 381-386.
15. Plaut, M., Pierce, J.H., Watson, C.J., Hanley-Hyde, J., Nordan, R.P., and Pau W.E. (1989). Mast cell lines produce lymphokines in response to cross-linkage of Fc RI or to calcium ionophores. Nature 339, 64-67.
16. Wodnar-Filipowicz, A., Heusser, C.H., and Moroni, C. (1989). Production of the haematopoietic growth factors GM-CSF and interleukin-3 by mast cells in response to IgE receptor-mediated activation. Nature 339, 150-152.
17. Steffen, M., Abboud, M., Potter, G.K., Yung, Y.P., and Moore, M.A.S. (1989). Presence of tumor necrosis factor or related factor in human basophil/mast cells. Immunology 66, 445-450.
18. Thueson, D.O., Speck, L.S., Lett-Brown, M.A., and Grant, J.A. (1979). Histamine releasing activity (HRA). I. Production by mitogen- or antigen-stimulated human mononuclear cells. J. Immunol. 123, 626-632.
19. Alam, R., Rozniecki, J., and Selmaj, K. (1984). A mononuclear cell-derived histamine releasing factor (HRF) in asthmatic

patients. Histamine release from basophils in vitro. Ann. Allergy 53, 66-69.
20. Schulman, E.S., Liu, M.C., Proud, D., MacGlashan, Jr, D.W., Lichtenstein, L.M, and Plaut, M. (1985). Human lung macrophages induce histamine release from basophils and mast cells. Am. Rev. Respir. Dis. 131, 230-235.
21. White, M.V, and Kaliner, M.A. (1987). Neutrophils and mast cells. I. Human neutrophil-derived histamine releasing activity. J. Immunol. 139, 1624-1630.
22. Orchard, M.A., Kagey-Sobotka, A., Proud, D., and Lichtenstein, L.M. (1986). Basophil histamine release induced by a substance from stimulated human platelets. J. Immunol. 136, 2240-2244.
23. Alam, R., Forsythe, P.A., Lett-Brown, M.A., and Grant, J.A. (1989). Cellular origin of histamine releasing factor (HRF) produced by mononuclear cells. J. Immunol. 142, 3951-3956.
24. Haak-Frendscho, M, Arai, N., Arai, K-I., Baeza, M.L., Finn, A., and Kaplari, A.P. (1988). Human recombinant granulocyte-macrophage colony stimulating factor and interleukin 3 cause basophil histamine release. J. Clin. Invest. 82, 17-20.
25. Alam, R., Welter, J.B., Forsythe, P.A., Lett-Brown, M.A., and Grant, J.A. (1989). Comparative effect of recombinant IL-1, -2, -3, -4, and -6, IFN-gamma, granulocyte-macrophage colony stimulating factor, tumor necrosis factor-alpha, and histamine-releasing factors on the secretion of histamine release from basophils. J. Immunol. 142, 3431-3435.
26. MacDonald, S., Schleimer, S.P., Kagey-Sobotka, A., Gillis, S., and Lichtenstein, L.M. (1989). Recombinant IL-3 induces histamine release from human basophils. J. Immunol. 142, 3527-3532.
27. Subramanian, N., and Bray, M.A. (1987). Interleukin 1 releases histamine from human basophils and mast cells in vitro. J. Immunol. 138, 271-275.
28. White, M.V., Yoshimura, T., Hook, W., Kaliner, M.A., and Leonard, E.J. (1989). Neutrophil attractant/activation protein-1 (NAP-1) causes human basophil histamine release. Immunol. Lett. 22, 151-154.
29. Massey W.A., Randall, T., MacDonald, S.M., Gillis, S., Allison, C., Kagey-Sobotka, A., and Lichtenstein, L.M. (1988). Recombinant human IL-1 enhances IgE-dependent basophil histamine release. Faseb J. 2, A1251 (abstr.).
30. Dahinden, C.A., Kurimoto, Y., De Weck, A., Lindley, I., Dewald, B., and Baggiolini, M. (1989). The neutrophil-activating peptide NAF/NAP-1 induces histamine release by interleukin 3-primed basophils. J. Exp. Med. 170, 1787-1792.
31. Schleimer, R.P., Derse, C.P., Friedman, B., Gillis, S., Plaut, M., Lichtenstein, L.M., and MacGlashan, Jr., D.W. (1989). Regulation of human basophil mediator release by cytokines. I. Interaction with antiinflammatory steroids. J. Immunol. 143, 1310-1317.

32. Kurimoto, Y., DeWeck, A.L., and Dahinden, C.A. (1989). Interleukin 3-dependent mediator release in basophils triggered by C5a. J. Exp. Med. 170, 467-479.
33. Baeza, M.L., Reddigari, S.R., Haak-Frendscho, M., Kornfeld, D., Gorevic, P.G., and Kaplan, A.P. (1988). Purification and characterization of human mononuclear cell histamine releasing factor. J. Clin. Invest. 83, 1204-1210.
34. Alam, R., Forsythe, P.A., Welter, J., Lett-Brown, M.A., and Grant, J.A. (1990). Purifcation of histamine releasing factor (HRF) produced by mononuclear cells and cell lines. J. Allergy Clin. Immunol. 85, 257 (abstr.).
35. Baeza, M.L., Reddigan, S.R., Kornfeld, D., Ramani, N., Smith, E.M., Hossler, P.A., Fischer, T., Castor, C.W., Gorevic, P.G., and Kaplan, A.P. (1990). Relationship of one of form of human histamine-releasing factor to connective tissue activating peptide-III. J. Clin. Invest. 85, 1516-1521.
36. Castor, C.W., Scott, R.M.E., and Whitney, S.L. (1977). Connective tissue activation. XI. Stimulation of glycosaminoglycan and DNA formation by a platelet factor. Arthritis Rheum. 20, 859-868.
37. Alam, R., Rozniecki, J., and Kuzminska, B. (1985). A lymphocyte-derived histamine releasing factor in bronchial asthma. III. Further studies. Ann. Allergy 55, 825-829.
38. Alam, R., Kuna, P., Rozniecki, J., and Kuzminska, B. (1987). The magnitude of spontaneous production of histamine releasing factor (HRF) by lymphocytes in vitro correlates with the state of bronchial hyperreactivity in patients with asthma. J. Allergy Clin. Immunol. 79, 103-108.
39. Kuna, P., Alam, R., Kuzminska, B., and Rozniecki, J. (1989). The effect of preseasonal immunotherapy on the production of histamine releasing factor (HRF) by mononuclear cells from patients with seasonal asthma. Results of a double-blind placebo-controlled randomized study. J. Allergy Clin. Immunol. 83, 816-824.
40. Kuna, P., Bochenska-Marciniak, M., Kuzminska, B., Rozniecki, J., and Alam, R. Stimulation of synthesis of histamine releasing factor(s) by mononuclear cells after allergen inhalation challenge of patients with asthma. (submitted for publication).
41. Warner, J.A., Pienkowski, M.M., Plaut, M., Norman, P.S, and Lichtenstein, L.M. (1986). Identification of histamine releasing factor(s) in the late phase of cutaneous IgE-mediated reactions. J. Immunol. 136, 2583-2587.
42. Hsieh, K-H., and Liao, T-N. (1990). Decreased production of and responsiveness to histamine-releasing factor after succesful immunotherapy in asthmatic children. J. Allergy Clin. Immunol. (in press).
43. MacDonald, S.M., Lichtenstein, L.M., Proud, D., Plaut, M., Naclerio, R.M., MacGlashan, D.W., and Kagey-Sobotka, A. (1987) Studies of IgE-dependent histamine releasing factors: heterogeneity of IgE. J. Immunol. 139, 506-512.

44. Alam, R., Forsythe, P.A., Rankin, J.A., Boyars, M.C., Lett-Brown, M.A., and Grant, J.A. Sensitivity of basophils to histamine releasing factor(s) of various orgin. Dependency on allergic phenotype of the donor and surface-bound IgE. J. Allergy Clin. Immunol. (in press).
45. Lichtenstein, L.M. (1988). Histamine releasing factors and IgE heterogeneity. J. Allergy Clin. Immunol. 81, 814-820.
46. Alam, R., Kuna, P., Rozniecki, J., and Kuzminska, B. (1986). Bacterial antigens stimulate the production of histamine releasing factor (HRF) by lymphocytes from intrinsic asthmatic patients. Clin. Exp. Immunol. 63, 241- 248.
47. Kuna, P., Alam, R., Rozniecki, J, and Kuzminska, B. (1988). The effect of autogenic bacterial antigens on the production of histamine releasing factor (HRF) by mononuclear cells from intrinsic asthmatic patients. Allergy 43, 511-518.
48. Alam, R., Grant, J.A., and Lett-Brown, M.A. (1988). Identification of a histamine release inhibitory factor produced by human mononuclear cells. J. Clin. Invest. 82, 2056-2062.
49. Leonard, E. J., and Yoshimura, T. (1990). Neutrophil attractant/activation protein-1 (NAP-1[interleukin-8]). Am. J. Respir. Cell Mol. Biol. 2, 479-486.
50. Gimbrone, Jr, M.A., Obin, M.S., Brook, A.F., Luis, E.A., Hass, P.E., Hebert, C.A., Yip, Y.K., Leung, D.W., Lowe, D.G., Kohr, W.J., Darbonne, W.C., Bechtol, K.B., and Baker, J.B. (1989). Endothelial interleukin-8: A novel inhibitor of leukocyte-endothelial interactions. Science 246, 1601-1603.
51. Alam, R., Welter, J., Forsythe, P.A., Lett-Brown, M.A., Rankin, J.A., Eoyars, M., and Grant, J.A. (1990). Detection of histamine release inhibitory factor- and histamine releasing factor-like activities in bronchoalveolar lavage fluids. Am. Rev. Respir. Dis. 141, 666-671.

AAS 31:
Mediators in
Airway Hyperreactivity

EFFECT OF LYMPHOKINES ON ß-ADRENOCEPTOR STIMULATION OF HUMAN PBMC

A.J.M. Van Oosterhout, W.B. Stam and F.P. Nijkamp

Department of Pharmacology, Faculty of Pharmacy, University of Utrecht, Catharijnesingel 60, 3511 GH Utrecht, The Netherlands

SUMMARY: The effect of IL-2, IL-3, IL-4 and GM-CSF on ß-adrenoceptor function of human peripheral blood mononuclear cells (PBMC) was studied. After a 2 h pre-incubation period of PBMC with each of the lymphokines (1-100 units/ml), the isoprenaline stimulated cAMP production in these cells was not altered. However, IL-2 and GM-CSF induced a concentration dependent decrease of the ß-adrenoceptor agonist stimulated cAMP production after a 20 h pre-incubation period.

INTRODUCTION

In asthma, a ß-adrenoceptor dysfunction may be the consequence of an active disease state rather than a fundamental abnormality as postulated by Szentivanyi (1968). It has been shown that in a guinea pig model of atopy in which the animals are injected intraperitoneally with bacterial endotoxin, the ß-adrenoceptor function of airway smooth muscle and of lymphocytes are decreased (Van Oosterhout et al., 1988a). This endotoxin-induced ß-adrenoceptor dysfunction can be prevented by splenectomy or by administration of the T-lymphocyte selective immunosuppressive drug cyclosporin-A (Van Oosterhout et al., 1988a,b). Based on these observations, it can be suggested that mediators produced by lymphocytes may be involved in ß-adrenoceptor dysfunction in this animal model. Since increasing evidence exists that T-lymphocytes are activated in acute severe asthma, mediators produced by these cells may also be involved in ß-adrenoceptor dysfunction in asthma (See Frew et al., 1990). To substantiate this hypothesis, we studied the influence of human interleukin-2 (IL-2), IL-3, IL-4 and granulocyte/macrophage colony stimulating factor (GM/CSF) on ß-adrenoceptor function of PBMC.

MATERIALS AND METHODS

PBMC were isolated from the blood of healthy volunteers or from buffy coats (Bloodbank, Utrecht, The Netherlands). Isolation was performed by centrifugation on a Ficoll-paque gradient (20 min, 1000 x g). Cells at the interface were removed and washed three times with RPMI-1640 (10 min, 500 x g). Finally, PBMC were suspended in RPMI-1640 at 3×10^7 cells/ml and pre-incubated without (control) or with IL-2 (Jurkat), IL-3, IL-4 and GM-CSF (all from Genzyme, Boston, USA). Pre-incubations were carried out at 37 °C in a humidified atmosphere of 5 % CO_2 / 95 % air. After a pre-incubation period of 2 or 20 h, 3×10^6 PBMC were incubated for 5 min at 37 °C in a shaking water bath, with or without 1 μM isoprenaline, in the presence of 0.5 mM 3-isobutyl-1-methyl-xanthine in a final volume of 200 μl. The reaction was terminated by means of heating the cell-suspensions in a boiling water bath for 5 min. Precipitated protein was centrifuged for 15 min at 1500 x g and 50 μl of the supernatant was used to measure cAMP content. cAMP was determined by a competitive protein binding method using a cAMP assay kit (Amersham, Great Britain)

RESULTS

Pre-incubation of PBMC with lymphokines during 2 or 20 h did not affect basal cAMP content of the cells as compared to control (results not shown).

Table: Isoprenaline induced cAMP production in human PBMC after pre-incubation with lymphokines during 20 h. Results are expressed as the percentage of the cAMP production by PBMC not incubated with lymphokine (control).

[Units/ml]	IL-2 (n=5)	IL-3 (n=5)	IL-4 (n=5)	GM-CSF (n=6)
Control	100.0 ± 21.3	100.0 ± 28.2	100.0 ± 21.3	100.0 ± 18.1
1	105.8 ± 8.8	104.3 ± 8.4	105.8 ± 10.7	95.5 ± 2.0
10	88.0 ± 8.5	96.0 ± 8.6	107.1 ± 20.3	88.2 ± 9.1
100	64.8 ± 7.6**	79.6 ± 14.1	97.6 ± 10.5	63.1 ± 10.7*

**: $P < 0.01$ and *: $P < 0.05$ as compared to control and determined with Student's paired t-test.

The increase in cAMP induced by the ß-adrenoceptor agonist isoprenaline (1 μM) was not changed when PBMC were pre-incubated with lymphokines during 2 h (results not shown). After a 20 h pre-incubation period, the isoprenaline-induced cAMP production was significantly decreased in PBMC incubated with IL-2 and GM-CSF at a concentration of 100 Units/ml (Table). The reduction of the ß-adrenoceptor agonist induced cAMP production amounted 35 ± 8 % ($P<0.01$, paired t-test) and 37 ± 11 % ($P<0.05$) in case of IL-2 and GM-CSF respectively. Pre-incubation of PBMC with IL-3 and IL-4 during 20 h did not influence ß-adrenoceptor function of the cells.

DISCUSSION

In the present study, we demonstrate that IL-2 and GM-CSF decrease ß-adrenoceptor agonist induced cAMP production in PBMC after a 20 h pre-incubation period. These results are in accordance with the data of Beckner & Farrar (1987) who demonstrated that IL-2 acutely decreases adenylate cyclase activity in activated human T-lymphocytes. In contrast to freshly isolated lymphocytes, activated lymphocytes express a large number of high affinity IL-2 receptors. This may explain that in our experiments the decreased ß-adrenoceptor function in PBMC only occurs after a 20 h and not after a 2 h pre-incubation period. GM-CSF is a T-lymphocyte glycoprotein that promotes the growth and differentiation of granulocytes and macrophages. It has been shown that GM-CSF (100 U/ml) acutely decreases adenylate cyclase activity in human neutrophils (Coffey et al., 1988). The inhibition of adenylate cyclase activity is maximal after 30 min pre-incubation, thereafter, the activity slowly recovers. In our experiments, no decreased isoprenaline-induced cAMP production is observed after 2 h pre-incubation of PBMC with GM-CSF (100 U/ml). However, when PBMC are incubated during 20 h with GM-CSF, the ß-adrenoceptor function is inhibited. An explanation for the delayed effect of GM-CSF can be that specific receptors have to be expressed on the cell membrane, analogous to IL-2 receptors.

In patients with asthma, it has been shown that dysfunction of the ß-adrenoceptor-adenylate cyclase complex occurs in leukocytes and airway smooth muscle (Lulich et al., 1988). Based on our findings, lymphokines may play a potential role in ß-adrenoceptor dysfunction in asthma. At present, little is known about the presence of lymphokine receptors on smooth muscle- and epithelial cells. Expression of IL-2 receptors was initially believed to be restricted to T-cells after their activation. However, it has been demonstrated that IL-2 receptor expression can be induced in B-lymphocytes, mast cells, monocytes and macrophages (Hancock et al., 1987). In previous experiments, we did not observe a decreased isoprenaline-induced relaxation of guinea pig tracheal spirals after 2 h pre-incubation with IL-2 (Van Oosterhout et al. 1990). More studies are needed to elucidate the effect of lymphokines on ß-adrenoceptor function of cells present in the respiratory airways.

ACKNOWLEDGEMENT

This study was supported by a research grant (87.29) of the Dutch Asthma Foundation.

REFERENCES

Beckner, S.K. and Farrar, W.L. (1987) Inhibition of adenylate cyclase by IL-2 in human T lymphocytes is mediated by protein kinase C. Biochem. Biophys. Res. Comm. 145, 176-182.

Coffey, R.G., Davis, J.S. and Djeu, J.Y. (1988) Stimulation of guanylate cyclase activity and reduction of adenylate cyclase activity by granulocyte-macrophage colony-stimulating factor in human neutrophils. J. Immunol. 140, 2695-2701.

Frew, A.J. and Kay, A.B. (1990) Eosinophils and T-lymphocytes in late-phase allergic reactions. J. Allergy Clin. Immunol. 85, 533-539.

Hancock, W.W., Muller, W.A. and Cotran, R.S. (1987) Interleukin 2 receptors are expressed by alveolar macrophages during pulmonary sarcoidosis and are inducible by lymphokine treatment of normal human lung macrophages, blood monocytes, and monocyte cell lines. J. Immunol. 138, 185-191.

Lulich, K.M., Goldie, R.G. and Paterson, J.W. (1988) Beta-adrenoceptor function in asthmatic bronchial smooth muscle. Gen. Pharmacol. 19, 307-311.

Szentivanyi, A. (1968) The beta-adrenergic theory of the atopic abnormality in bronchial asthma. J. Allergy Clin. Immunol. 42, 203-220.

Van Oosterhout, A.J.M., Folkerts, G., Ten Have, G.A.M. and Nijkamp, F.P. (1988a) Involvement of the spleen in the endotoxin-induced deterioration of the respiratory airway and lymphocyte ß-adrenergic systems of the guinea pig. Eur. J. Pharmacol. 147, 421-430.

Van Oosterhout, A.J.M., Woutersen-Van Nijnanten, F.M.A. and Nijkamp, F.P. (1988b) Cyclosporin A prevents endotoxin-induced ß-adrenoceptor impairment in lymphocytes. Eur. J. Pharmacol. 149, 191-192.

Van Oosterhout, A.J.M. and Nijkamp, F.P. (1990) Effect of human interleukin-2 from different sources on lymphocyte and airway ß-adrenoceptor function. Int. J. Immunopharmacol. 12, 409-412.

AAS 31:
Mediators in
Airway Hyperreactivity

A ROLE FOR T CELLS IN THE INDUCTION OF AIRWAY HYPERREACTIVITY

J. Garssen[1,2], H. Van Loveren[2], H. Van Der Vliet[1], H. Bot[2], F.P. Nijkamp[1]

[1]Faculty of Pharmacy, Department of Pharmacology, University of Utrecht, The Netherlands, and [2]National Institute of Public Health and Environmental Protection, Bilthoven, The Netherlands.

SUMMARY: In this study we investigated a possible relationship of delayed type hypersensitivity (DTH), as a model for cellular IgE-independent immunity, with the induction of airway hyperreactivity. In PCl (picryl chloride) sensitized BALB/c mice DTH-like lung infiltrates were found that were maximal 48 hr after intranasal hapten challenge. During the elicitation of this DTH-like reaction tracheal hyperreactivity to the cholinergic agonist carbachol could be detected from 2 hr after challenge with the homologous hapten and that was maximal after 48 hr.

INTRODUCTION

A common denominator of almost all asthmatics is an increased reactivity of the airways to nonspecific stimuli (airway hyperreactivity). The underlying mechanisms are still unknown. An array of inflammatory cells and their mediators are denoted as possible candidates to contribute to the induction of airway hyperresponsiveness (Postma et al., 1989). An important cell type that is thought to be involved in asthma is the mast cell (Holgate, 1989). Mediators released by mast cells could play an important role in asthma-like diseases. There is now substantial evidence that antigen-specific T-cell factors are capable of activating mast cells to release mediators (Meade et al., 1988;

Van Loveren et al., 1987). This in contrast to IgE dependent mast cell degranulation or mast cell degranulation induced by non-specific stimuli like pseudoallergens. In this study we investigated whether a T cell/mast cell interaction, as occurs in the initiation phase of DTH could play a role in the induction of airway hyperreactivity.

MATERIALS AND METHODS

Sensitization and challenge procedure: BALB/c mice were skin-sensitized with PCl and challenged intranasally with a water soluble form of PCl (i.e. PSA,picryl sulfonic acid) 7 days later as described elsewhere (Garssen et al., 1989). Non-sensitized control mice were challenged similarly.

Detection of inflammatory responses: At various time points after challenge lungs were removed and filled intratracheally with fixative for histological studies (Garssen et al., 1989). Additional two days after challenge lungs were lavaged and cell counts were performed using a haemocytometer. We characterized the percentage of cell subtypes (pan-T cells, $L3T4^+$-T cells, $Ly2^+$-T cells, IgM^+ cells, moma-1 and moma-2 cells, and @-$asialo^+$cells), from cell populations made by enzymatic digestion of whole lungs, using a Becton Dickinson FACS-scan.

Determination of tracheal reactivity: Determination of tracheal reactivity to carbachol was performed as described elsewhere at several time points after challenge of sensitized or non-sensitized mice (Garssen et al., 1990). For comparing specific curve parameters the cumulative dose response curves were analyzed and the EC50 values for each individual curve were calculated. The EC50 values were subsequently averaged for the various groups and differences in EC50 values (=ΔEC50) were determined and statistically tested using the unpaired Student's t-test.

RESULTS

In this study we have confirmed and extended studies from Enander et al. (1985) and found a pulmonary reaction in PCl sensitized mice that were challenged intranasally with the homologous hapten. The reaction was maximal 48 hr after challenge and could be detected histologically (Garssen et al, 1989) but also using cell counts in bronchoalveolar lavages. The cell counts from lung lavages from sensitized and challenged mice ($12.6 \pm 0.9 \times 10^5$ cells) differed significantly ($p<0.001$) from non-sensitized mice ($5.4 \pm 0.3 \times 10^5$ cells). The majority of these cells were macrophages but also T cells (maximal 30 %) could be detected. Using cell populations made from whole lungs we found that the percentage of the lymphoid cell subtypes that we have tested, were similar except for a small but statistically significant increase in the percentage of $L3T4^+$-T cells (T-help cells)(table I).

Table I: Percentage of subpopulations of lymphoid cells in murine lung

	non-sensitized, PSA challenged mice (n=11)	PCl sensitized, PSA challenged mice (n=11)	
L3T4*	8.5±1.03	13.4±1.69	$p<0.05$
Ly2*	8.7±1.51	10.6±1.42	
Thyl.2*	22.7±1.06	22.3±2.08	
IgM*	27.9±2.75	28.4±1.96	
momal**	1.0±0.36	2.1±0.72	
moma2**	10.0±1.24	11.1±1.78	
@-asialo***	51.8±2.47	52.8±1.27	

*L3T4, Ly2, Thyl.2, and IgM are monoclonal antibodies that recognize respectively T-help cells, T-suppressor or T-cytotoxic cells, pan-T cells, and B cells.
**momal and moma2 are monoclonal antibodies that recognize subpopulations of certain macrophages/monocytes (Kraal et al., 1986,1987).
***asialo antibodies recognize natural killer cells and monocytes

Tracheas from PSA challenged mice, sensitized 1 week earlier, showed a significant hyperreactivity to carbachol as compared to challenged non-sensitized control mice. This hyperreactivity was especially characterized by a shift of the dose-response curve to the left, indicating a decreased EC50. The maximal decrease of the EC50 value was found 48 hr after challenge (table II).

Table II: Differences in EC50 values at various time points after challenge

time after PSA challenge	$\Delta EC50 \cdot 10^{-7}$	*
2 hours	3.7	$p<0.02$
24 hours	2.8	$p<0.01$
48 hours	5.7	$p<0.001$
72 hours	3.3	$p<0.02$
96 hours	1.8	$p<0.01$
3 weeks	-0.1	n.s.

*ΔEC50 is the averaged EC50 value of non-sensitized mice minus the averaged EC50 value of sensitized mice (n=5-6 for each group at each time point).

DISCUSSION AND CONCLUSION

We have studied induction of airway hyperreactivity by lung DTH, as a model for cellular IgE-independent immunity and found an increased tracheal reactivity to carbachol in sensitized mice that was maximal 48 hr after challenge. This hyperreactivity could already be detected 2 hr after challenge. Two hours after challenge we did not find an inflammatory reaction but we could detect increased vascular permeability that is serotonin dependent (Garssen et al., 1989). Although we cannot rule out that the DTH-like infiltrate, that was characterized by an infiltrate of mononuclear cells (especially L3T4 cells), influenced the ultimate reactivity to carbachol, hyperreactivity to this cholinergic agonist did not depend on the actual presence of the infiltrate. The data suggest therefore that T cell dependent steps in the initiation of DTH could be responsible for the induction of airway hyperreactivity. The model that we present here, and that describes a role for cell mediated immunity in the induction of airway hyperreactivity may shed light on those forms of asthma in which IgE does not seem to play a predominant role, such as the case in occupational asthma induced by small molecular weight substances like isocyanates and chromium salts (O'Byrne et al., 1987; Olaguibel et al., 1989).

Acknowledgements: We are grateful to Dr. G. Kraal (Free University, Amsterdam) for the gift of moma1 and moma2 antibodies.

REFERENCES

Enander, I., Ahlstedt, S., and Nygren, H. (1986). Cyclophosphamide-mediated enhancement of delayed hypersensitivity reactions in the lung. Int. Archs. Allergy Appl. Immun. 79, 291-295.

Garssen, J., Nijkamp, F.P., Wagenaar, Sj.Sc., Zwart, A., Askenase, P.W., and Van Loveren, H. (1989). Regulation of delayed-type hypersensitivity-like responses in the mouse lung, determined with histological procedures: Serotonin, T cell suppressor inducer factor, and high antigen dose tolerance regulate the magnitude of T cell dependent inflammatory reactions. Immunology 68, 51-58.

Garssen, J., Van Loveren, H., Van Der Vliet, H., and Nijkamp, F.P. (1990). An isometric method to study respiratory smooth muscle responses in mice. J. of Pharm. Methods, in press.

Holgate, S.T. (1989). Mast cell activation in asthma. Agents Actions Suppl. 28, 57-66.

Kraal, G., and Janse, M. (1986). Marginal metallophilic cells of the mouse spleen identified by a monoclonal antibody. Immunology 58, 665-669.

Kraal, G., Rep, M., and Janse, M. (1987). Macrophages in T and B cell compartments and other tissue macrophages recognized by monoclonal antibody moma-2. An Immunohistochemical Study. Scan. J. Immunol. 26, 653-661.

Meade, R., Van Loveren, H., Parmentier, H., Iverson, M., and Askenase, P.W. (1988). The antigen-binding T cell factor PCl-F sensitizes mast cells for in vitro release of serotonin. J. Immunol. 141, 2704-2713.

O'Byrne, P.M., Dolovich, J., and Hargreave, F.E. (1987). Late asthmatic responses. Am. Rev. Resp. Dis. 136, 740-751.

Olaguibel, J.M., and Basomba, A. (1989). Occupational asthma induced by chromium salts. Allergol. Immunopathol. 17, 133-136.

Postma, D.S., Koëter, G.H., and Sluiter, H.J. (1989). In: Airway responsiveness and atopy in the development of chronic lung disease (S.T. Weiss, and D. Sparrow, Eds.), Raven Press , New York, 2, pp. 21-71.

Van Loveren, H., Ptak, W., and Askenase, P.W. (1987). Involvement of antigen specific T cell factors in regulation of separate steps in the DTH cascade. Lymphokines 14,405-429.

AAS 31:
Mediators in
Airway Hyperreactivity

NEUROPEPTIDES AS MODULATORS OF AIRWAY FUNCTION

Peter J Barnes

Department of Thoracic Medicine, National Heart and Lung Institute, Brompton Hospital, London SW3 6LY, UK.

SUMMARY: Many neuropeptides have recently been identified in human and animal airways. These peptides, which may coexist with classical transmitters, have potent effects on airway calibre, blood vessels and secretions, raising the possibility that they may be involved in airway diseases such as asthma. Vasoactive intestinal peptide and peptide histidine methionine have potent relaxant effects on both vascular and bronchial smooth muscle, and may be neurotransmitters of non-cholinergic vasodilatation and non-adrenergic bronchodilation. Several neuropeptides which are found in sensory nerves, such as substance P, neurokinin A and calcitonin gene-related peptide, have both direct inflammatory effects and influence inflammatory cells, and might also contribute to the pathology of asthma if released from sensory nerve endings by an axon reflex.

INTRODUCTION

The distribution and potent effects of neuropeptides on various aspects of airway function suggest that they may be involved in controlling airway smooth muscle, blood flow, vascular permeability and mucus secretion (Uddman α Sundler, 1987; Barnes, 1987b). Asthma, which is characterised by airway hyperreresponsiveness of the airways, was attributed to abnormal nervous mechanisms until the middle of the present century, when immunological and mediator theories of pathogenesis gained favour. The demonstration of an extensive network of nerve fibres containing potent peptides, in addition to classical neurotransmitters, in the airways has revived interest in possible neural abnormalities in asthma. Recent experimental and clinical studies suggest that asthma and bronchial hyperreactivity may be associated with an inflammatory response in the airway wall. Neural and neuropeptide control mechanisms might be involved in, as well as influenced by, this airway inflammation.

Neural control of airways is far more complex than previously recognised (Barnes, 1986a). In addition to the classical cholinergic and adrenergic mechanisms, neural pathways which are neither adrenergic nor cholinergic (NANC) have been described. Both excitatory (bronchoconstrictor) and inhibitory (bronchodilator) NANC mechanisms have been described in airways of animals and humans (Anderson & Grundstrom, 1983; Barnes, 1986a). NANC nerves also regulate tracheo-bronchial vascular resistance and blood flow (Widdicombe, 1990), microvascular leakage (Lundberg et al, 1983b), and mucus secretion (Peatfield & Richardson, 1983). The physiological role of these nervous pathways is likely to remain obscure until specific blockers become available, however.

It was once believed that neuropeptides were localised to their own "peptidergic" nerves in airways, but it is increasingly apparent that neuropeptides occur as cotransmitters within classical adrenergic, cholinergic and sensory nerves and may interact with these nerves in a complex way.

VASOACTIVE INTESTINAL PEPTIDE

Effects on tracheo-bronchial smooth muscle: Vasoactive intestinal peptide (VIP), a 28 amino acid peptide, is the neuropeptide found in highest concentrations in human lung and is localised to efferent nerves (Uddman & Sundler, 1987; Lundberg et al, 1984a). VIP-immunoreactive nerve fibres are associated with airway smooth muscle (particularly in large airways), mucus glands, airway blood vessels and parasympathetic ganglia (which contain VIP-immunoreactive nerve cell bodies). VIP relaxes human bronchi *in vitro* and is almost 100-fold more potent than isoprenaline, making it the most potent endogenous bronchodilator so far discovered (Palmer et al, 1986a). In asthmatic patients nebulised VIP is rather disappointing, since it has no bronchodilator effect and provides only weak protection against histamine-induced bronchospasm, probably because little of the nebulised peptide can reach receptors in airway smooth muscle (Barnes & Dixon, 1984). VIP similarly has no bronchodilator effect when infused in normal subjects (who bronchodilate with isoprenaline), probably because the profound hypotensive and vasodilator effects of the peptide limit the dose which can be given in human subjects (Palmer et al, 1986b).

VIP is the most favoured candidate for the neurotransmitter

of NANC inhibitory nerves since in animal airways it mimics the electrophysiological changes produced by NANC nerve stimulation (Cameron et al, 1983), it is released when these nerves are stimulated electrically (Matsuzaki et al, 1980), and when tolerance is induced by exposure to high concentrations of VIP, the NANC inhibitory nerve effects (but not sympathetic inhibitory effects) are reduced (Ito α Takeda, 1982). Furthermore, both the bronchodilator action of VIP and inhibitory NANC effects are potentiated by a type III phosphodiesterase inhibitor (Rhoden α Barnes, 1990a).

Histochemical studies show that VIP-immunoreactive nerves diminish in the smaller airways and are virtually absent from bronchioles (Lundberg et al, 1984a). Autoradiographic mapping of VIP-receptors has demonstrated that, while smooth muscle of large airways has VIP-receptors, they are absent for smooth muscle of peripheral airways (Carstairs α Barnes, 1986a). Interestingly, non-adrenergic relaxation, evoked by electrical field stimulation, is almost absent in small airways and these airways fail to relax with VIP, although isoprenaline is effective (Palmer et al, 1986a). Taken together, the evidence points towards VIP as a neurotransmitter of NANC inhibitory nerves but certain proof must await the development of specific receptor antagonists.

Other airway effects: In animals, VIP is also a potent stimulant of airway mucus secretion (Peatfield et al, 1983), and of fluid transport across airway epithelium (Nathanson et al, 1983), suggesting that VIP-ergic nerves may also regulate airway secretions. VIP is a very potent vasodilator and, in the tracheal circulation, might play an important role in regulation of perfusion of the airways (Laitinen et al, 1987). It is more potent as a vasodilator in the tracheal than the bronchial circulation (Matran et al, 1989), and may mediate the vasodilator response to vagus nerve stimulation in upper airways.

Autoradiographic mapping of VIP-receptors in human and guinea-pig lung has confirmed the presence of receptors on airway glands, epithelium and vascular smooth muscle (Carstairs α Barnes, 1986a). Vascular smooth muscle appears to have the highest density of VIP-receptors, in agreement with the demonstration that VIP is a potent vasodilator.

Cotransmission with acetylcholine: Electron microscopic studies have indicated that VIP may be present in cholinergic nerves in the airways, and may therefore function as a co-transmitter with acetylcholine (Laitinen et al, 1985b). VIP reduces the contractile effect of acetylcholine on airway smooth muscle *in vitro* and may therefore act as a "braking" mechanism to cholinergic bronchoconstriction (Barnes, 1987a). It is possible that VIP is co-released only under certain patterns of neural activation, such as high frequency firing, thus acting as a protective mechanism. Another possible physiological role for VIP could involve regulation of local blood flow. If cholinergic nerve activity causes bronchoconstriction, release of VIP from activated cholinergic nerves may have an effect on nearby vessels, so that blood flow increases as smooth muscle contracts, thus supplying more nutrients to active smooth muscle cells under metabolic demand (Barnes, 1987b).

<u>Peptide histidine methionine</u>: Peptide histidine isoleucine (PHI) is a 27 amino acid with marked structural similarities to VIP and is coded by the same gene. In humans there is a terminal methionine, giving the name peptide histidine methionine (PHM). PHI/PHM is present in the same nerves as VIP (Lundberg et al, 1984a) and has rather similar effects. PHM is equipotent to VIP as a relaxant of airway smooth muscle (Palmer et al, 1986a), although is less potent as a vasodilator than VIP, suggesting that it might act on different receptors, or have a different rate of degradation. Peptide histidine valine (PHV-42) is a precursor of VIP and is also a potent bronchodilator <u>in vitro</u> (Yiangou et al, 1987), but whether it is released from airway nerves is still unknown. Like VIP, it has no effect on airway function in human subjects (Chilvers et al, 1988).

<u>Inhibitory NANC nerves and asthma</u>: Whether any abnormality in inhibitory NANC nerves or VIP might contribute to airway hyperresponsiveness is uncertain. NANC-inhibitory nerves have been demonstrated in human airways <u>in vitro</u> by electrical field stimulation (Barnes, 1986a) and, in the absence of demonstrable

sympathetic bronchodilator nerves, this is the only neural bonchodilator mechanism. NANC bronchodilator nerves have also been demonstrated in normal human subjects in vivo by a variety of means (Michoud et al, 1987; Lammers et al, 1988; Ichinose et al, 1988). However, in mild asthmatics there is no apparent defect in this neural bronchodilator pathway (Lammers et al, 1989). However, it is possible that abnormal function of NANC bronchodilator nerves only becomes apparent in more severe asthma, when there is presumably a greater degree of inflammation. A defect in the inhibitory control of airway smooth muscle tone would certainly account for some of the features of airway hyperrsponsiveness. A striking absence of VIP-immunoreactive nerves has been described in patients with severe asthma (Ollerenshaw et al, 1989a). Inflammatory cells identified in the asthmatic airway, such as neutrophils, eosinophils and mast cells may release a variety of peptidases which would rapidly break down VIP and PHM. Indeed, VIP is a good substrate for mast cell tryptase (Caughey et al, 1988). Rapid degradation of the inhibitory cotransmitter VIP may be like taking the brake off cholinergic nerves, resulting in exaggerated reflex cholinergic bronchoconstriction, at least in proximal airways. While this is unlikely to be the primary cause of asthma it could contribute to the airway hyperresponsiveness associated with airway inflammation.

PEPTIDES IN SENSORY NERVES

Substance P: Substance P (SP) is localised to unmyelinated

sensory nerves (C-fibres) in airways (Uddman & Sundler, 1987; Lundberg et al, 1984b), and has several affects which are reminiscent of the inflammatory response of asthma. SP exerts its effects on target cells via specific receptors, which have been localised by autoradiography to smooth muscle of all airways, from trachea to small bronchioles, and therefore it may regulate the caliber of peripheral airways (Carstairs & Barnes, 1986b). In addition to contraction of airway smooth muscle, SP also potently stimulates mucus secretion from submucosal glands and goblet cells (Coles et al, 1984; Rogers et al, 1990; Barnes et al, 1990a). SP potently increases airway microvascular permeability and exudation of plasma into the airway lumen (Lundberg et al, 1983b; Rogers et al, 1989) and vasodilates tracheo-bronchial circulation (Matran et al, 1989). SP also degranulates mast cells of the skin (Foreman et al, 1983), although this has not been demonstrated conclusively in lung, and may have chemotactic effects on inflammatory cells.

Non-cholinergic bronchoconstrictor nerves have been demonstrated *in vitro* and *in vivo* in guinea-pigs (Anderson & Grundstrom, 1983). These nerves are antagonised by an SP antagonist (Lundberg et al, 1983b), suggesting that SP or a related tachykinin may be the excitatory neurotransmitter. These studies raise the possibility that SP might be released from sensory nerve endings by an axon reflex mechanism.

Capsaicin, the hot extract of pepper, releases SP from unmyelinated sensory nerve endings and, in rats and guinea-pigs, this pungent agent causes acute bronchoconstriction and airway microvascular leakiness (Lundberg et al, 1987). Capsaicin also releases SP and other peptides from perfused guinea pig lung (Saria et al, 1988). Chronic treatment with capsaicin leads to depletion of SP-immunoreactivity and other tachykinins as well as CGRP (see below) and can, therefore, be used as a tool to investigate the contribution of peptides in C-fibre afferent nerves to airway responses. Depletion of peptides from sensory nerves is associated with a reduced vasodilator response to allergen in sensitised animals (Lundberg et al, 1987; Alving et al, 1988), and prevents irritants, such as cigarette smoke or mechanical stimulation of the airway, from causing airway microvascular leakage (Lundberg α Saria, 1983).

While these local effects of SP innervation are clearly demonstrable in rodents, the relevance of these findings to human airways is less certain. Reports of SP innervation of human airways are conflicting (Laitinen et al, 1983; Lundberg et al, 1984b), but human lungs obtained at surgery are usually from older smokers in whom SP content may be reduced. A preliminary report suggests that SP-immunoreactive nerves may be increased in the airways of patients with severe asthma, however (Ollerenshaw et al, 1989b). SP causes contraction of human airways in vitro, and capsaicin causes similar contraction, suggesting the release of SP from nerves within airway smooth muscle (Lundberg et al, 1983a). Inhalation of capsaicin in human volunteers also causes bronchoconstriction, although this is only transient and may be due to a laryngeal reflex (Fuller et al, 1985). Inhalation of SP has no effect (Fuller et al, 1987c), even in asthmatic patients, presumably because the peptide is metabolised by airway epithelial cells and is not able to reach receptors on bronchial smooth muscle.

Other tachykinins: A related peptide, neurokinin A (NKA) has also been isolated from the mammalian nervous system, and is found in the same airway nerves that contain SP (Martling et al, 1987). SP and NKA appear to activate different tachykinin receptors. NKA is far more potent than SP in contracting airway smooth muscle (Martling et al, 1987; Advenier et al, 1987; Palmer α Barnes, 1987), suggesting that the receptors on airway smooth muscle are of the NK-2 type. By contrast, SP is more potent than NKA as a bronchial vasodilator and in causing airway microvascular leakage (Rogers et al, 1989; McCormack et al, 1988), indicating that NK-1 receptors are present on the vasculature. SP is also more potent than NKA in stimulating mucus secretion from human bronchi and from airway goblet cells, indicating that NK-1 receptors regulate airway secretions (Rogers et al, 1988; Barnes et al, 1990b). Nebulised and infused NKA, but not SP, also causes bronchoconstriction in asthmatic patients (Fuller et al, 1987c; Joos et al, 1987; Evans et al, 1988). NKA also facilitates cholinergic neurotransmission in guinea pig airways and would thus tend to exaggerate cholinergic reflex bronchoconstriction (Hall et al, 1989).

Another mammalian tachykinin, neurokinin B, appears to activate a third receptor subtype (NK-3 receptor), but NKB has not yet been identified in airway nerves (Martling et al, 1987); a fourth tachykinin receptor has also been proposed in guinea-pig trachea (McKnight et al, 1989), but does not appear to be present on human bronchi (Rhoden α Barnes, 1990b).

Role of epithelium: Airway epithelium modulates the bronchoconstrictor effect of many spasmogens, possibly by releasing a relaxant substance similar to endothelium-derived relaxant factor. This is particularly relevant in asthma, since airway epithelium may be shed or damaged even in mild asthmatics. Epithelium removal markedly potentiates the bronchoconstrictor effect of tachykinins (Grandordy et al, 1988). For NKA this can be explained by the fact that the major metabolising enzyme for tachykinins, neutral endopeptidase (enkephalinase) is localised to airway epithelium (Sekizawa et al, 1987). Inhibition of this enzyme by specific inhibitors, such as phosphoramidon or thiorphan, potentiates bronchoconstriction to the same extent as epithelial removal (Frossard et al, 1989). For SP it is more complex, since SP also appears to release relaxant factors from airway epithelium via NK-1 receptors on epithelial cells (Frossard et al, 1989). Thus, if epithelium is shed in asthma the tachykinins released from sensory nerves in the airways are likely to have much more pronounced effects, not only on bronchoconstriction but also on microvascular leakage and mucus secretion.

Calcitonin gene-related peptide: Another peptide which has recently been localised to sensory nerves is calcitonin gene-related peptide (CGRP), which may also be co-stored and co-released with SP (Lundberg et al, 1985). CGRP has no consistent effects on guinea pig airways (Martling et al, 1988) but contracts human airways _in vitro_ (Palmer et al, 1987), although perhaps a more important effect is in regulation of airway blood flow, since it produces intense and long-lasting vasodilation in skin (Fuller et al, 1987a). It is also a potent vasodilator of bronchial vessels both _in vivo_ and _in vitro_ (Salonen et al, 1988; McCormack et al, 1989). Receptor mapping studies have shown that CGRP-receptors are localised predominantly to bronchial vessels in animal and human airways (Mak α Barnes, 1988), further suggesting that CGRP may be an important regulator of bronchial blood flow, perhaps contributing to the hyperaemic appearance of asthmatic airways. CGRP does not cause microvascular leakage in airways (Rogers et al, 1988), but theoretically could increase the leakage produced by other agents. CGRP potentiates the leakage produced by SP in skin, but this does not occur in airways, possibly because blood flow is higher than in skin (Rogers et al, 1988).

Neurogenic inflammation in asthma: Because neuropeptides like SP, NKA and CGRP mimic many of the inflammatory features of asthma it is tempting to speculate that they may be involved in its pathogenesis, and the idea of neurogenic inflammatory mechanisms in asthma is attractive (Barnes, 1986b; Barnes, 1990). Damage to airway epithelium may occur even in relatively mild asthmatics, thereby exposing afferent nerve endings (Laitinen et al, 1985a). These nerve endings may then be stimulated by inflammatory mediators in the airway lumen. Bradykinin, an inflammatory peptide formed by enzymatic cleavage from a plasma precursor, is likely to be found in the asthmatic airway by the action of enzymes released from inflammatory cells on exuded plasma. Bradykinin selectively stimulates C-fibre nerve endings (Kaufman et al, 1980) and may release sensory neuropeptides (Saria et al, 1988). Bradykinin is a potent bronchoconstrictor in asthmatic patients (Fuller et al, 1987b) and may result in the release of sensory neuropeptides such as SP, NKA and CGRP from collateral branches of sensory nerves, via an axon reflex. This could result in bronchoconstriction, mucus hypersecretion and microvascular leakage leading to oedema of the airway wall and extravasation of plasma in the lumen. Furthermore, epithelial shedding would lead to loss of neutral endopeptidase so that any tachykinins released would have a greater effect (Frossard et al, 1989). Axon reflexes may then amplify the inflammatory response and may spread inflammatory changes in the airway mucosa from patchy areas of epithelial damage. It follows that therapies which reduce axon reflex mechanisms might prove to be beneficial in asthma.

Modulation of neurogenic inflammation: Several drugs appear to modulate the release of sensory neuropeptides from sensory nerves (Barnes et al, 1990a). Opioids, which inhibit the release of SP in the CNS, are also very effective in inhibiting NANC bronchoconstriction, both in vitro and in vivo (Frossard α Barnes, 1987; Belvisi et al, 1988) and airway neurogenic microvascular leakage (Belvisi et al, 1989b), acting via u-opioid receptors on sensory nerve endings. Recent evidence suggests that the inhibitory neurotransmitter gamma-aminobutyric acid (GABA) acting via GABA B-receptors may also inhibit tachykinin release from airway sensory nerves (Belvisi et al, 1989a). Neuropeptide Y and galanin are also effective. Cromoglycate is an anti-asthma drug whose mode of action is unknown. It is remarkably effective in reducing the dyspnoea and bronchoconstriction due to inhaled bradykinin in asthmatic patients (Fuller et al, 1987a; Dixon α Barnes, 1989), suggesting that it may prevent activation of sensory nerves. This is in agreement with early experimental studies which demonstrated that cromoglycate reduced the firing of airway C-fibres (Dixon et al, 1979).

OTHER NEUROPEPTIDES

Several other neuropeptides have been identified in human airway nerves, although their physiological role is far from certain.

Neuropeptide Y: Neuropeptide Y (NPY) is a cotransmitter in

adrenergic nerves of the lung. It may play a role in regulating bronchial blood flow and modulation of airway ganglia, rather than airway smooth muscle directly, since sympathetic nerves are relatively sparse in airway smooth muscle in humans. Recent studies suggest that NPY may modulate cholinergic and NANC neurotransmission in airways (Stretton α Barnes, 1988; Matran et al, 1989b), as in well as reducing tracheal blood flow (Salonen et al, 1988).

Cholecystokinin: Cholecystokinin octapeptide (CCK8) has been found in lung in low concentrations. CCK8 is a potent constrictor of proximal human and guinea-pig airways in vitro, acting directly on receptors in airway smooth muscle. These receptors are potently antagonised by the peripheral CCK antagonist L 363,851, indicating that they may belong to the CCK-A receptor type (Stretton α Barnes, 1989).

CCK8 does not appear to influence either ganglionic transmission or postganglionic cholinergic nerves in guinea-pig. The constrictor effect of CCK-8 is enhanced by epithelium removal and by phosphoramidon, suggesting that, like tachykinins, it is metabolised by neutral endopeptidase in airway epithelium (Stretton α Barnes, 1989). Interestingly, the responses to CCK are similarly enhanced in sensitised animals after exposure to allergen, which is presumably explained by epithelial dysfunction.

CONCLUSIONS

There has been an explosion of knowledge about the effects of neuropeptides in animal and human airways, yet we still know very little about the physiological role of these peptides in the regulation of airway function, and even less about their role in airway diseases such as asthma. This information will only come with the development of specific antagonists for neuropeptides. Although there has been some progress, the development of peptide antagonists is beset by problems in clinical practice because of instability or difficulty in delivery to target cell receptors. Non-peptide antagonists would be preferable but progress has been slow.

The ultimate goal of research into airway neuropeptides is to provide new approaches to therapy. Perhaps the most fruitful area may be in pursuing drugs which inhibit the release of multiple neuropeptides via prejunctional receptors on sensory nerve endings. Such drugs could be expected to have a beneficial action in asthma by reducing neurogenic inflammation.

Acknowledgement: I am very grateful to Madeleine Wray for her careful preparation of the manuscript.

REFERENCES

Advenier, C., Naline, E., Drapean, G., and Regoli, D. (1987). Relative potencies of neurokinins in guinea-pig and human bronchus. Eur J Pharmacol. 139: 133-137.

Alving, K., Matran, R., Lacroix, J.S., and Lundberg, J.M. (1988). Allergen challenge induces vasodilatation in pig bronchial circulation via a capsaicin sensitive mechanism. Acta Physiol Scand. 134: 571-572.

Andersson, R.G.G., and Grundstrom, N. (1983). The excitatory non-cholinergic, non-adrenergic nervous system of the guinea-pig airways. Eur J Respir Dis. 64 (Suppl 121): 141-157.

Barnes, P.J. (1986a). State of Art. Neural control of human airways in health and disease. Am Rev Respir Dis. 134: 1289-1314.

Barnes, P.J. (1986b). Asthma as an axon reflex. Lancet. i: 242-245.

Barnes, P.J. (1987a). Airway neuropeptides and asthma. Trends Pharm Sci. 8: 24-27.

Barnes, P.J. (1987b). Neuropeptides in the lung: localization, function and pathophysiologic implications. J Allergy Clin Immunol. 79: 285-295.

Barnes, P.J. (1990). Neurogenic inflammation in airways and its modulation. Arch int Pharmacodyn. 303: 67-82.

Barnes, P.J., Belvisi, M.G. and Rogers, D.F. (1990a). Modulation of neurogenic inflammation: novel approaches to inflammatory diseases. Trends Pharmacol Sci. 11: 185-189.

Barnes, P.J., and Dixon, C.M.S. (1984). The effect of inhaled vasoactive intestinal peptide on bronchial hyperreactivity in man. Am Rev Respir Dis. 130: 162-166.

Barnes, P.J., Kuo, H.P., Rogers, D.F., Rohde, J.A.L. and Tokuyama, K. (1990b). Effect of sensory neuropeptides on goblet cell secretion in guinea pig trachea <u>in vivo</u>. J Physiol. 422: 99P.

Belvisi, M.G., Chung, K.F., Jackson, D.M., and Barnes, P.J. (1988). Opioid modulation of non-cholinergic neural bronchoconstriction in guinea-pig <u>in vivo</u>. Br J Pharmacol. 95: 413-418.

Belvisi, M.G., Ichinose, M. and Barnes, P.J. (1989a). Modulation of non-adrenergic non-cholinergic neural bronchoconstriction in guinea-pig airways via GABA-B receptors. Br J Pharmacol. 97: 1125-1131.

Belvisi, M.G., Rogers, D.F., and Barnes, P.J. (1989b). Neurogenic plasma extravasation: inhibition by morphine in guinea pig airways in vivo. J Appl Physiol. In press.

Cameron, A.R., Johnston, C.D., Kirkpatrick, C.T., and Kirkpatrick, M.C.A. (1983). The quest for the inhibitory neurotransmitter in bovine tracheal smooth muscle. Q J Exp Psychol. 68: 413-426.

Carstairs, J.R., and Barnes, P.J. (1986a). Visualization of vasoactive intestinal peptide receptors in human and guinea pig lung. J Pharmacol Exp Ther. 239: 249-255.

Carstairs, J.R., and Barnes, P.J. (1986b). Autoradiographic mapping of substance P receptors in lung. Eur J Pharmacol. 127: 295-296.

Caughey, G.H., Leidig, F., Viro, N.F., and Nadel, J.A. (1988). Substance P and vasoactive intestinal peptide degradation by mast cell tryptase and chymase. J Pharmacol Exp Ther. 244: 133-137.

Chilvers, E.R., Dixon, C.M.S., Yiangou, Y., Bloom, S.R., and Ind, P.W. (1988). Effect of peptide histidine valine on cardiovascular and respiratory function in normal subjects. Thorax. 43: 750-755.

Coles, S.J., Neill, K.H., and Reid, L.M. (1984). Potent stimulation of glycoprotein secretion in canine trachea by substance P. J Appl Physiol. 57: 1323-1327.

Dixon, C.M.S., and Barnes, P.J. (1989). Bradykinin induced bronchoconstriction: inhibition by nedocromil sodium and sodium cromoglycate. Br J Clin Pharmacol. 27: 831-836.

Dixon, M., Jackson, D.M., and Richards, I.M. (1979). The effect of sodium cromoglycate on lung irritant receptors and left ventricular receptors in anaesthetised dog. Br J Pharmacol. 67: 569-574.

Evans, T.W., Dixon, C.M.S., Clarke, B., Conradson, T.-.B., and Barnes, P.J. (1988). Comparison of neurokinin A and substance P on cardiovascular and airway function in man. Br J Clin Pharmacol. 25: 273-275.

Foreman, J.C., Jordan, C.C., Oehme, P., and Renner, H. (1983). Structure-activity relationships for some substance P-related peptides that cause wheal and flare reactions in human skin. J Physiol. 335: 449-465.

Frossard, N., and Barnes, P.J. (1987). u-Opioid receptors modulate non-cholinergic constrictor nerves in guinea-pig airways. Eur J Pharmacol. 141: 519-522.

Frossard, N., Rhoden, K.J., and Barnes, P.J. (1989). Influence of epithelium on guinea pig airway responses to tachykinins: role of endopeptidase and cyclooxygenase. J Pharmacol Exp Ther. 248: 292-298.

Fuller, R.W., Dixon, C.M.S., and Barnes, P.J. (1985). The bronchoconstrictor response to inhaled capsaicin in humans. J Appl Physiol. 85: 1080-1084.

Fuller, R.W., Conradson, T.-.B., Dixon, C.M.S., Crossman, D.C. and Barnes, P.J. (1987a). Sensory neuropeptide effects in human skin. Br J Pharmacol. 92: 781-788.

Fuller, R.W., Dixon, C.M.S., Cuss, F.M.C., and Barnes, P.J. (1987b). Bradykinin-induced bronchoconstriction in man: mode of action. Am Rev Respir Dis. 135: 176-180.

Fuller, R.W., Maxwell, D.L., Dixon, C.M.S., McGregor, G.P., Barnes, V.F., Bloom, S.R., and Barnes, P.J. (1987c). The effects of substance P on cardiovascular and respiratory function in human subjects. J Appl Physiol. 62: 1473-1479.

Grandordy, B.M., Frossard, N., Rhoden, K.J., and Barnes, P.J. (1988). Tachykinin-induced phosphoinositide breakdown in airway smooth muscle and epithelium: relationship to contraction. Mol Pharmacol. 33: 515-519.

Hall, A.K., Barnes, P.J., Meldrum, L.A., and Maclagan, J. (1989). Facilitation by tachykinins of neurotransmission in guinea-pig pulmonary parasympathetic nerves. Br J Pharmacol. 97: 274-280.

Ichinose, M., Inoue, H., Miura, M., and Takishima, T. (1988). Nonadrenergic bronchodilation in normal subjects. Am Rev Respir Dis. 138: 31-34.

Ito, Y., and Takeda, K. (1982). Non-adrenergic inhibitory nerves and putative transmitters in the smooth muscle of cat trachea. J Physiol. 330: 497-511.

Joos, G., Pauwels, R., and van der Straeten, M. (1987). Effect of inhaled substance P and neurokinin A on the airways of normal and asthmatic subjects. Thorax. 42: 779-783.

Kaufman, M.P., Coleridge, H.M., Coleridge, J.C.G., and Baker, D.G. (1980). Bradykinin stimulates afferent vagal

C-fibres in intrapulmonary airways of dogs. J Appl Physiol. 48: 511-517.

Laitinen, L.A., Heino, M., Laitinen, A., Kava, T., and Haahtela, T. (1985a). Damage of the airway epithelium and bronchial reactivity in patients with asthma. Am Rev Respir Dis. 131: 599-606.

Laitinen, L.A., Laitinen, A., Panula, P.A., Partanen, M., Tervo, K. and Tervo, T. (1983). Immunohistochemical demonstration of substance P in the lower respiratory tract of the rabbit and not of man. Thorax. 38: 531-536.

Laitinen, L.A., Laitinen, A., Salonen, R.O., and Widdicombe, J.G. (1987). Vascular actions of airway neuropeptides. Am Rev Respir Dis. 136: S59-64.

Laitinen, A., Partanen, M., Hervonen, A., Peto-Huikko, M., and Laitinen, L.A. (1985b). VIP-like immunoreactive nerves in human respiratory tract. Light and electron micrsoscopic study. Histochemistry. 82: 313-319.

Lammers, J.-.W., Minette, P., McCusker, M.T., Chung, K.F., and Barnes, P.J. (1988). Nonadrenergic bronchodilator mechanisms in normal human subjects in vivo. J Appl Physiol. 64: 1817-1822.

Lammers, J.-.W., Minette, P., McCusker, M.T., Chung, K.F. and Barnes, P.J. (1989). Capsaicin-induced bronchodilation in asthmatic patients: role of the nonadrenergic inhibitory system. J Appl Physiol. 67: 856-861.

Lundberg, J.M., Anders, F.-.C., Hua, X., Hokfelt, T., and Fischer, J.A. (1985). Coexistence of substance P and calcitonin gene-related peptide-like immunoreactivities in sensory nerves in relation to cardiovascular and bronchoconstrictor effects of capsaicin. Eur J Pharmacol. 108: 315-319.

Lundberg, J.M., Fahrenkrug, J., Hokfelt, T., Martling, C.-.R., Larsson, O., Tatemoto, K., and Anggard, A. (1984a). Coexistence of peptide H1 (PH1) and VIP in nerves regulating blood flow and bronchial smooth muscle tone in various mammals including man. Peptides. 5: 593-606.

Lundberg, J.M., Hokfelt, T., Martling, C.-.R., Saria, A., and Cuello, C. (1984b). Substance P-immunoreactive sensory nerves in the lower respiratory tract of various mammals including man. Cell Tissue Res. 235: 251-261.

Lundberg, J.M., Martling, C.-.R., and Saria, A. (1983a). Substance P and capsaicin-induced contraction of human bronchi. Acta Physiol Scand. 119: 49-53.

Lundberg, J.M., and Saria, A. (1983). Capsaicin-induced desensitization of the airway mucosa to cigarette smoke, mechanical and chemical irritants. Nature. 302: 251-253.

Lundberg, J.M., Saria, A., Brodin, E., Rusells, S., and Folkers, R. (1983b). A substance P antagonist inhibits vagally induced increase in vascular permeability and bronchial smooth muscle contraction in the guinea-pig. Proc Nat Acad Sci. 80: 1120-1124.

Lundberg, J.M., Saria, A., Lundblad, L., Angaard, A., Martling, C.-.R., Theodorsson-Norheim, E., Stjarne, P., and Hokfelt, T. (1987). Bioactive peptides in capsaicin-sensitive

C-fibre afferents of the airways: functional and pathophysiological implications. In: The Airways: Neural Control in Health and Disease. Kaliner MA, Barnes PJ, eds. New York: Marcel Dekker. pp 417-445.

Mak, J.C.M., and Barnes, P.J. (1988). Autoradiographic localization of calcitonin gene-related peptide binding sites in human and guinea pig lung. Peptides. 9: 957-964.

Martling, C.-.R., Saria, A., Fischer, J.A., Hokfelt, T., and Lundberg, J.M. (1988). Calcitonin gene-related peptide and the lung: neuronal coexistence with substance P, release by capsaicin and vasodilatory effect. Regul Pept. 20: 125-139.

Martling, C.-.R., Theordorsson-Norheim, E., and Lundberg, J.M. (1987). Occurrence and effects of multiple tachykinins: substance P, neurokinin A, neuropeptide K in human lower airways. Life Sci. 40: 1633-1643.

Matran, R., Alving, K., Martling, C.-.R., Lacroix, J.S., and Lundberg, J.M. (1989a). Vagally mediated vasodilation by motor and sensory nerves in the tracheal and bronchial circulation of the pig. Acta Physiol Scand. 135: 29-37.

Matran, R., Martling, C.-.R., and Lundberg, J.M. (1989b). Neuropeptide Y and alpha2-receptor inhibition of cholinergic and non-adrenergic, non-cholinergic bronchoconstriction. Eur J Pharmacol. In press.

Matsuzaki, Y., Hamasaki, Y., and Said, S.I. (1980). Vasoactive intestinal peptide: a possible transmitter of nonadrenergic relaxation of guinea pig airways. Science. 210: 1252-1253.

McCormack, D.G., Salonen, R.O. and Barnes, P.J. (1989). Effect of sensory neuropeptides on canine bronchial and pulmonary vessels <u>in vitro</u>. Life Sci. 45: 2405-2412.

McKnight, A.T., Maguire, J.J., Varney, M.A., and Williams, B.J. (1989). Characterization of receptors for tachykinins using selectivity of agonists and antagonists: evidence for an NK-4 receptor in guinea-pig isolated trachea. J Physiol. 409: 30.

Michoud, M.-.C., Amyot, R., Jeanneret-Grosjean, A., and Couture, J. (1987). Reflex decrease of histamine-induced bronchoconstriction after laryngeal stimulation in humans. Am Rev Respir Dis. 136: 618-622.

Nathanson, I., Widdicombe, J.H., and Barnes, P.J. (1983). Effect of vasoactive intestinal peptide on ion transport across dog tracheal epithelium. J Appl Physiol. 55: 1844-1848.

Ollerenshaw, S., Jarvis, D., Woolcock, A., Sullivan, C. and Scheibner, T. (1989a). Absence of immunoreactive vasoactive intestinal polypeptide in tissue from the lungs of patients with asthma. N Engl J Med. 320: 1244-1248.

Ollerenshaw, S.L., Jarvis, D.L., Woolcock, A.J., Scheibner, T. and Sullivan, C.E. (1989b). Substance P immunoreactive nerve fibres in airways from patients with and without asthma. Am Rev Respir Dis. 139: 237.

Palmer, J.B.D., and Barnes, P.J. (1987). Neuropeptides and airway smooth muscle function. Am Rev Respir Dis. 136: S50-54.

Palmer, J.B., Cuss, F.M.C., and Barnes, P.J. (1986a). VIP

and PHM and their role in non-adrenergic inhibitory responses in isolated human airways. J Appl Physiol. 61: 1322-1328.

Palmer, J.B.D., Cuss, F.M.C., Mulderry, P.K., Ghatei, M.A., Springall, D.R., Cadieux, A., Bloom, S.R., Polak, J.M., and Barnes, P.J. (1987). Calcitonin gene-related peptide is localised to human airway nerves and potently constricts human airway smooth muscle. Br J Pharmacol. 91: 95-101.

Palmer, J.B.D., Cuss, F.M.C., Warren, J.B., and Barnes, P.J. (1986b). The effect of infused vasoactive intestinal peptide on airway function in normal subjects. Thorax. 41: 663-666.

Peatfield, A.C., Barnes, P.J., Bratcher, C., Nadel, J.A., and Davis, B. (1983). Vasoactive intestinal peptide stimulates tracheal submucosal gland secretion in ferret. Am Rev Respir Dis. 128: 89-93.

Peatfield, A.C., and Richardson, P.S. (1983). Evidence for non-cholinergic, non-adrenergic nervous control of mucus secretion into the cat trachea. J Physiol. 342: 335-345.

Rhoden, K.J. and Barnes, P.J. (1990a). Potentiation of non-adrenergic non-cholinergic relaxation in guinea pig airways by a cAMP phosphodiesterase inhibitor. J Pharmacol Exp Ther. 282: 396-402.

Rhoden, K.J. and Barnes, P.J. (1990b). Classification of tachykinin receptors on guinea-pig and human airway smooth muscle. Am Rev Respir Dis. 141: A726.

Rogers, D.F., Belvisi, M.G., Aursudkij, B., Evans, T.W., and Barnes, P.J. (1988). Effects and interactions of sensory neuropeptides on airway microvascular leakage in guinea pigs. Br J Pharmacol. 95: 1109-1116.

Rogers, D.F., Aursudkij, B. and Barnes, P.J. (1989). Effects of tachykinins on mucus secretion in human bronchi <u>in vitro</u>. Eur J Pharmacol. 174: 283-286.

Salonen, R.O., Webber, S.E., and Widdicombe, J.G. (1988). Effects of neuropeptides and capsaicin on the canine tracheal vasculature <u>in vivo</u>. Br J Pharmacol. 95: 1262-1270.

Saria, A., Martling, C.-.R., Yan, Z., Theordorson-Norheim, E., Gamse, R., and Lundberg, J.M. (1988). Release of multiple tachykinins from capsaicin-sensitive sensory nerves in the lung by bradykinin, histamine, dimethylphenyl piperazinium and vagal nerve stimulation. Am Rev Respir Dis. 137: 1330-1335.

Sekzizawa, K., Tamaoki, J., Graf, P.D., Basbaum, C.B., Borson, D.B. and Nadel, J.A. (1987). Enkephalinase inhibitor potentiates mammalian tachykinin-induced contraction in ferret trachea. J Pharmacol Exp Ther. 243: 1211-1217.

Stretton, D., and Barnes, P.J. (1988). Modulation of cholinergic neurotransmission in guinea-pig trachea by neuropeptide Y. Br J Pharmacol. 93: 672-678.

Stretton, C.D., and Barnes, P.J. (1989). Cholecystokinin octapeptide constricts guinea-pig and human airways. Br J Pharmacol. 97: 675-682.

Uddman, R., and Sundler, F. (1987). Neuropeptides in the airways: a review. Am Rev Respir Dis. 136: S3-8.

Widdicombe, J.G. (1990). The NANC system and airway vasculature. Arch int Pharmacodyn. 303: 83-90.

Yiangou, Y., Di Marzo, V., Spokes, R.A., Panico, M., Morris,

H.R. and Bloom, S.R. (1987). Isolation, characterization, and pharmacological actions of peptide histidine valine 42, a novel prepro-vasoactive intestinal peptide-derived peptide. J Biol Chem. 262: 14010-14013.

AAS 31:
Mediators in
Airway Hyperreactivity

MODULATION OF CHOLINERGIC NEUROTRANSMISSION BY VIP, VIP-ANTISERUM AND VIP-ANTAGONISTS IN DOG AND CAT TRACHEA: VIP PLAYS A ROLE OF "DOUBLE BRAKING" IN BRONCHO-CONSTRICTION

Y. Ito and H. Hakoda

Department of Pharmacology, Faculty of Medicine, Kyushu University, Fukuoka 812, Japan

SUMMARY: Exogeous VIP in low concentrations has a prejunctional action inhibiting the excitatory neuroeffector transmission in addition to a direct inhibitory action on the smooth muscle cells, by suppressing transmitter release from the vagus nerve terminals in dog and cat trachea. In the cat trachea, effects of VIP antiserum and VIP antagonists indicate that endogenous VIP may contribute to non-adrenergic non-cholinergic inhibitory response and inhibits acetylcholine (ACh) release from the vagus nerve terminals. Endogenous VIP may play a "double braking" role in broncho-constriction in the cat trachea.

INTRODUCTION

Parasympathetic nervous system in the airways involves inhibitory neurotransmitters in addition to ACh. These are neither adrenergic nor cholinergic (NANC) in nature, but neuropeptides such as VIP, PHI or PHM are candidates as possible neurotransmitters (Ito & Takeda, 1982, Ellis & Farmer, 1989 a & b). VIP-immunoreactive nerves was localized to cholinergic nerves, and ultrastructual studies have demonstrated the presence of peptidergic granules within cholinergic nerves in the airway smooth muscle (Latinen et al., 1985a). Thus, VIP and ACh may co-exist in the same nerve terminals (Lundberg, 1981), and VIP may be released as a co-transmitter (Barnes, 1986). Then, a simple question arises as to the physiological meaning of the co-existence of excitatory and inhibitory neurotransmitters in the same nerve terminals.

To make a clue to this question, we analyzed the effects of VIP, VIP-antiserum and VIP-antagonists on the contractions and excitatory junction potentials (EJPs) recorded from dog and cat trachea.

MATERIALS AND METHODS

Segments of cervical trachea were excised from adult mongrel dogs (10-13 kg) and cats (2-3 kg), and a dorsal strip of transversely running smooth muscle was separated from the cartilage. The tracheal smooth muscle was cut a width of 2.0-2.5 mm, 4-5 mm or 1-2 mm and a length of 8-10 mm, 10-15 mm or 1-2 mm for the double sucrose-gap, microelectrode and isometric tension recording methods, respectively. The preparation was bathed in a modified Krebs solution. The double sucrose-gap method was used to record the membrane potential and tension development of the tissue as described elsewhere (Ito & Tajima, 1981). For intracellular recording of the membrane potential, a conventional microelectrode filled with 3M-KCl (30-50MΩ) was inserted from outer surface of the preparation. To produce neurogenic responses, electrical field stimulation (50 μs in duration and about 10-20V in strength) was applied. The following drugs were used: vasoactive intestinal polypeptide (VIP; Peptide Institute, Osaka), rabbit antiporcine VIP antiserum, non-immune serum from a non-immunized rabbit (Funakoshi, Tokyo), VIP antagonists, [Ac-Tyr^1, D-Phe$_2$]-GRF(1-29)-NH_2 and [4-Cl-D-Phe^6, Leu^{17}]-VIP (Cosmo. Bio., Tokyo).

RESULTS

VIP(10^{-11}-10^{-7}M) dose-dependently reduced the amplitude of the contractions evoked by field stimulation in the combined presence of indomethacin (10^{-5}M) and guanethidine (10^{-6}M) in the dog, and in the presence of guanethidine (10^{-6}M) in case of cat trachea. In parallel with actions on twitch contractions, VIP (10^{-11}-10^{-7}M) reduced the amplitude of EJPs evoked by single pulse field stimulation in both tissues. VIP (10^{-11}-10^{-9}M) had no effect on the post-junctional sensitivity to exogenous ACh, on the resting membrane potential or on the input resistance of the smooth muscle cells of dog and cat trachea, indicating that low concentrations of VIP (10^{-11}-10^{-9}M) act prejunctionally to inhibit excitatory neuroeffector transmission, presumably by supressing ACh from the vagus nerves.

During repetitive field stimulation at the stimulus frequency of 0.033-0.1 Hz, the amplitude of the EJPs was gradually reduced (the depression), and VIP (10^{-9}M) enhanced this depression phenomenon in the dog and cat trachea. EJPs also showed summation when repetitive field stimulation was applied at high frequency (20 Hz), and the slope of the relationship between the relative amplitude of EJPs and number of stimuli at 20 Hz was 2.2±0.4 mV/stimulus in the dog trachea. However, in the cat trachea, summation of EJPs was not prominent, giving a mean slope of 0.6±0.02 mV/stimulus measured by the micro-electrode. VIP (10^{-9}M) shifted downward the relationship between the relative amplitude of EJPs and number of stimuli at 20 Hz in both tissues. Overnight incubation with VIP-antiserum (10^{-6}g/ml) markedly reduced amplitude of the muscle relaxation in the cat trachea and had little effect on the depression of EJPs in the dog and cat trachea, or the summation of the EJPs observed in the dog trachea. However, this procedure markedly enhanced the summation of EJPs observed in the cat trachea, and the mean slope of the relationship between relative amplitude of EJPs and number of stimuli at 20 Hz was increased from 0.6±0.2 to 1.5±0.1 mV/stimulus. The VIP antagonists, [Ac-Tyr^1, D-Phe^2]-GRF(1-29)-NH_2(>10^{-9}M) and [4-Cl-D-Phe^6, Leu^{17}]-VIP(>10^{-8}M), dose-dependently increased the amplitude of the EJPs in the cat trachea when a single stimulus was applied with no change in the membrane potential and input membrane resistance. Overnight incubation of the cat tracheal tissue with [4-Cl-D-Phe^6, Leu^{17}]-VIP(10^{-7}M) enhanced the summation of EJPs evoked by repetitive field stimulation at 20 Hz.

DISCUSSION

In ferret trachea, it was reported that VIP has a dual effects on cholinergic neurotransmission at different concentrations (facilitation up to 10^{-9}M VIP and inhibition at 10^{-8}-$2x10^{-7}$M VIP), probably through a specific VIP receptor (Sekizawa et al., 1988). The present results indicate that low concentration of VIP (10^{-11}-10^{-9}M) act prejunctionally to inhibit excitatory neuroeffector transmission by suppressing ACh release from the vagus nerves in the dog and cat trachea, in addition to the well documented direct inhibitory actions on the airway smooth muscle cells. Enhancement of the depression of EJPs by VIP, and inhibitory effects of VIP on the summation of EJPs observed in the dog and cat tracheal tissue also support the presynaptic actions of VIP on the cholinergic nerve terminals.

One of the most prominent difference in the property of EJPs observed in the dog and cat tracheal tissues is the summation phenomenon. When several stimuli at 20 Hz were applied, a linear relationship between the number of stimuli and the amplitude of the EJPs was observed in the dog, but this was not the case in the cat trachea. After treatment with VIP

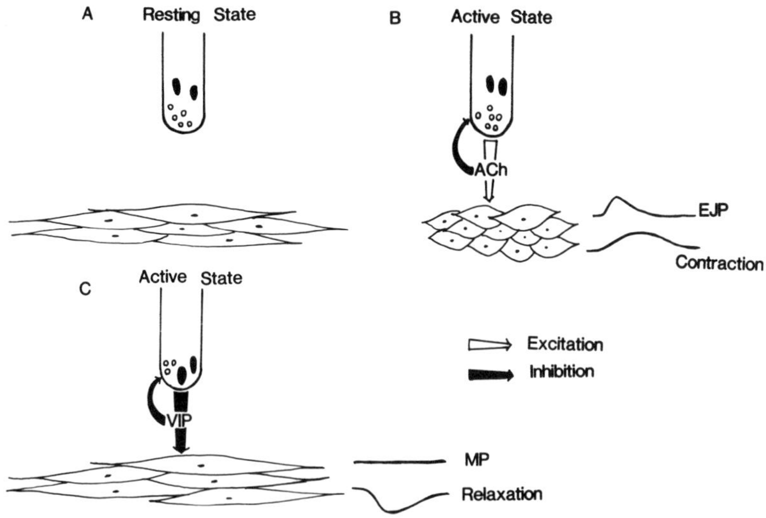

Fig.1. Postulated effects of endogenous VIP on neuroeffector transmission in the cat trachea. ACh released from the vagus nerve terminal evokes EJP and following contraction, and reduces the effect of vagus nerve activity (B, see Ito & Yoshitomi 1988). Endogenous VIP relaxes the muscle and also reduces the effect of vagus nerve activity especially when higher stimulus frequencies were employed (C).

antiserum, EJPs recorded from the cat trachea showed summation in response to repetitive field stimulation at 20 Hz, giving mean slopes of 1.1±0.4 mV/stimulation and 1.5±0.1 mV/stimulation measured by double sucrose-gap and microelectrode methods. Furthermore, VIP antagonists enhanced the amplitude of the EJPs within 5-10 min, and overnight incubation with [4-Cl-D-Phe^{6}, Leu^{17}]-VIP markedly enhanced the summation phenomenon of EJPs of the cat trachea evoked by repetitive field stimulations. The question of whether VIP is the neurotransmitter of NANC nerves in the cat airways has yet to be answered. However, if VIP does serve as a neurotransmitter it may play an important role in inhibiting ACh release from the vagus nerve terminal in addition to the well-known direct relaxing action on the smooth muscle cells, thus playing a "double braking" role in broncho-constriction (Fig. 1.). Lung tissues obtained at autopsy or lobectomy from subjects, with or without asthma, have been examined for immunoreactivity to VIP, and it turned out that the specimens from asthmatic patients did not show immunoreactivity to VIP (Ollerenshaw et al., 1989). This indicates that in patients with asthma there is a loss of VIP from pulmonary nerve fibres and this loss may diminish neurologically mediated bronchodilatation. ACh is one of the most potent agents causing broncho-constriction, and the parasymapathetic nerves are the dominant broncho-constrictor neural pathways. Such being the case, the overactivity of cholinergic mechanisms may contribute to bronchial hyper-responsiveness (Nadel et al., 1986), and the modulatory mechanisms may play an important role related to cholinergic broncho-constriction.

REFERENCES

Barnes, P.J. (1986). Neural control of human airways in health and diseases. Am. Rev. Resp. Disease, 134, 1289-1314.

Ellis, J.L. & Farmer, S.G. (1989a). Effects of vasoactive intestinal peptide (VIP) antagonists, VIP and peptide histidine isoleucine antisera on non-adrenergic, non-cholinergic relaxations of tracheal smooth muscle. Brit. J. Pharmacol., 96, 513-520.

Ellis, J.L. & Farmer, S.G. (1989b). Effects of peptidases on non-adrenergic, non-cholinergic inhibitory responses of tracheal smooth muscle: a comparison with effects on VIP- and PHI-induced relaxation. Brit. J. Pharmacol., 96, 521-526.

Ito, Y. & Tajima, K. (1981). Actions of indomethacin and prostaglandins on neuro-effector transmission in the dog trachea. J. Physiol., 319, 379-392.

Ito, Y. & Takeda, K. (1982). Non-adrenergic inhibitory nerves and putative transmitters in the smooth muscle of cat trachea. J. Physiol., 330, 499-511.

Ito, Y. & Yoshitomi, T. (1986). Autoregulation of acetylcholine release from vagus nerve terminals through activation of muscarinic receptors in the dog trachea. Br. J. Pharmacol., 93, 636-646.

Lundberg, J.M. (1981). Evidence for coexistence of vasoactive intestinal polypeptide (VIP) and acetylcholine in neurone of cat exocrine glands. Acta. Physiol. Scand. Suppl., 496, 1-57.
Nadel, J.A., Barnes, P.J. & Holtzman, M.J. (1986). Autonomic factors in the hyper-reactivity of airway smooth muscle. In handbook of Physiology; Respiratory System (3) pp. 693-702. American Physiological Society. Washington, D.C., U.S.A.
Ollerenshaw, S., Jarvis, D., Woolcock, A., Sullivan, C.,& Scheibner, J. (1989). Absence of immunoreactive vasoactive intestinal polypeptide in tissue from the lungs of patients with asthma. New Engl. J. Med., 320, 1244-1248.
Sekizawa, K., Tamaoki, J., Graf, P.D. & Nadel, J.A. (1988). Modulation of cholinergic neurotransmission by vasoactive intestinal peptide in ferret trachea. J. Appl. Physiol., 64, 2433-2437.

AAS 31:
Mediators in
Airway Hyperreactivity

CHARACTERISATION OF THE NEUROKININ RECEPTORS MEDIATING CONTRACTION OF ISOLATED TRACHEAL PREPARATIONS FROM A VARIETY OF SPECIES

R.L.G. Sheldrick, D.I. Ball and R.A. Coleman

Peripheral Pharmacology Department, Glaxo Group Research Ltd., Ware, Herfordshire, SG12 0DP, U.K.

SUMMARY: The effects of neurokinin (NK) agonists on isolated tracheal preparations from rat (RT), pig (PT), rabbit (RbT) and guinea-pig (GPT) have been investigated. None of the NKs contracted RT, suggesting that this preparation lacks NK receptors mediating contraction, whereas NKs caused concentration- related contractions of PT, RbT and GPT. In PT, NK_1-receptors mediate contraction since only substance P (SP) and the NK_1-receptor selective agonists, SP methylester (SPOMe) and GR73632 were highly potent. In contrast, in RbT, only NKA and the selective NK_2-receptor agonist, GR64349 were potent, indicating the presence of NK_2-receptors. However, in GPT both NK_1- and NK_2-receptors appear to mediate contraction to NKs since NKA, GR73632 and GR64349 were highly potent and SP and SPOMe moderately potent agonists. This study demonstrates apparent species differences in the NK-receptor populations present in tracheal smooth muscle.

INTRODUCTION

Neurokinins (NKs) contract human bronchial smooth muscle, an action which appears to be mediated by NK_2-receptors (Advenier et al., 1987; Dion et al., 1990). NKs also contract airway smooth muscle from other species: in guinea-pig trachea (GPT) this effect is mediated by both NK_1- and NK_2-receptors (Devillier et al., 1988; Ireland et al., 1988, 1990) whereas in hamster trachea, only NK_2-receptors appear to be involved (Maggi et al., 1989). In the present study, we have investigated the contractile effects of NKs on isolated tracheal preparations from a wider range of species, including rat (RT), pig (PT), rabbit (RbT) as well as guinea-pig. The results of these studies provide a clear indication of the NK-receptors present in each of these preparations.

METHODS

Tracheas were removed from male rats (AHA strain), male neonatal pigs (large whites, 3-10 days old), rabbits of either sex (New Zealand Whites) and male guinea-pigs (Dunkin-Hartley). Tracheal strips (2-3 cartilage rings thick) were prepared as described by Coleman (1987). The lumen of the tracheal strip was rubbed with a moist cotton wool bud to remove the epithelium, an effect which was confirmed histologically. Tracheal strips were mounted in organ baths in oxygenated Krebs solution (see Coleman, 1987) at $37^{o}C$. The Krebs solution contained indomethacin (2.8μM), atropine, mepyramine, methysergide (all at 1μM) and the peptidase inhibitors, phosphoramidon (1μM) and bestatin (100μM).

Cumulative concentration-effect curves were obtained to substance P (SP), neurokinin A (NKA), neurokinin B (NKB), the selective NK_1-receptor agonists SP methylester (SPOMe) and GR73632 (δ-aminovaleryl[$LPro^9$,N-$MeLeu^{10}$]SP(7-10)), the selective NK_2-receptor agonist, GR64349 ([Lys^3,Gly^8-R- -lactam-Leu^9]NKA(3-10)) and the selective NK_3-receptor agonist, senktide (see Ireland et al., 1988; Hagan et al., 1989).

RESULTS

In the RT preparation, NKA, NKB, SPOMe, GR64349 and senktide, in the concentration range 0.01-10μM, were all devoid of contractile activity, whereas carbachol (1-300μM) caused concentration-related contractions.

On the PT, SP and the NK_1-receptor selective agonists, SPOMe and GR73632, were all potent, contractile agonists, with EC_{50} values in the range 5-15nM. NKA was also moderately potent, being only 10-fold weaker than SP. However, NKB and the more selective NK_2- and NK_3-receptor agonists, GR64349 and senktide respectively, although still causing contractile responses, were more than 100-fold weaker than SP (see Figure 1).

In the RbT, NKA and the selective NK_2-receptor agonist, GR64349 were the most potent contractile agonists, with EC_{50} values of 4-6nM. Of the other NKs, only NKB, SP and GR73632 had marked contractile activity, but were between 90 and 1000-fold less potent than NKA. The selective NK_1- and NK_3-receptor agonists, SPOMe and senktide respectively, were virtually inactive (see Figure 1).

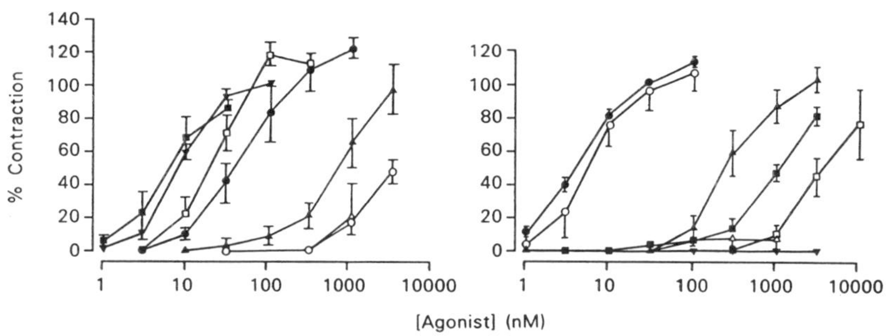

Figure 1: Mean concentration-effect curves to SP (■), NKA (●), NKB (▲), SPOMe (▼), GR73632 (□), GR64349 (o) and senktide (Δ) on pig trachea (left panel) and rabbit trachea (right panel). On the ordinate, 100% is an arbitary value given to the contractile response obtained to SPOMe (100nM) in pig trachea and NKA (30nM) in rabbit trachea, all other responses being expressed as a percentage of this response. Each point is the mean of at least 4 independent determinations, vertical bars represent s.e.mean.

On GPT, like RbT, NKA and the selective NK_2-receptor agonist, GR64349 were potent contractile agonists, with EC_{50} values of approximately 3nM. However, on this preparation, SP and the selective NK_1-receptor agonists, GR73632 and SPOMe, also had appreciable agonist activity, being between 4 and 20-fold less potent than NKA. The NK_3-receptor selective agonist, senktide was more than a 1000-times weaker than NKA.

The results obtained with NKs on these different tracheal preparations are summarized in Table I.

Table I The contractile potency of neurokinins on tracheal smooth muscle from a range of species

Agonist	PT (SP EC_{50} = 4.7 [2.5-8.9]nM)	GPT (NKA EC_{50} = 3.0 [1.4-6.6]nM)	RbT (NKA EC_{50} = 4.1 [3.2-5.3]nM)	RT
	Equipotent concentration ratio (most potent agonist = 1)			
SP	1.0 (0.5-2.2)	19[a]	198 (101-386)	NT
NKA	10 (6-17)	1.0 (0.6-1.7)	1.0[a]	Inactive[b]
NKB	122 (72-203)	72 (29-177)	89 (22-358)	Inactive[b]
SPOMe	1.7[a]	20 (11-38)	>3000	Inactive[b]
GR73632	3.3 (1.5-7.2)	4.1 (1.5-11)	1010 (260-3960)	NT
GR64349	352 (168-735)	1.0 (0.2-7.3)	1.5 (0.4-5.7)	Inactive[b]
Senktide	>140	>1000	>135	Inactive[b]

Values are geometric means (95% C.L.) $n \geq 4$, [a] = standard agonist, [b] = tested at 0.01-10μM, NT = not tested

DISCUSSION

The results of the present study confirm the presence of contractile NK-receptors in GPT, and indicate that such receptors are also present in both PT and RbT. No evidence for the presence of contractile NK-receptors was obtained in RT. It is not clear at present whether relaxant NK-receptors exist in any of these preparations, and further experiments will be required to investigate this possibility. As to the nature of the NK-receptors in these various tracheal preparations, the results obtained support the previous suggestion that GPT contains a mixed NK_1/NK_2 population (Ireland et al., 1990). In contrast, the results demonstrate only NK_1-receptors in PT and only NK_2-receptors in RbT.

This study has therefore shown that there are species differences in the NK-receptors mediating contraction of tracheal smooth muscle. While the present results give some indication as to the nature of the NK-receptor populations present in guinea-pig, pig and rabbit trachea, confirmation of these findings awaits the use of selective NK-receptor blocking drugs.

REFERENCES

Advenier, C., Naline, E., Drapeau, G. and Regoli, D. (1987). Relative potencies of neurokinins in guinea-pig trachea and human bronchus. Eur. J. Pharmacol. 139, 133-137.

Coleman, R.A. (1987). Methods in prostanoid receptor classification. In: Benedetto, C. et al (eds) Prostaglandins and related substances, a practical approach. IRL Press, Oxford, 267-303.

Devillier, P., Advenier, C., Drapeau, G., Marsac, J. and Regoli, D. (1988). Comparison of the effects of epithelium removal and of an enkephalinase inhibitor on the neurokinin-induced contractions of guinea-pig isolated trachea. Br. J. Pharmacol., 94, 675-684.

Dion, S., Rouissi, N., Nantel, F., Drapeau, G., Regoli, D., Naline, E. and Advenier, C. (1990). Receptors for neurokinins in human bronchus and urinary bladder are of the NK_2 type. Eur. J. Pharmacol., 178, 215-219.

Hagan, R.M., Ireland, S.J., Jordan, C.C., Bailey, F., Stephens-Smith, M., Deal, M. and Ward, P. (1989). Novel, potent and selective agonists at NK_1- and NK_2-receptors. Br. J. Pharmacol., 98, 717P.

Ireland, S.J., Jordan, C.C., Stephens-Smith, M. and Ward, P. (1988). Receptors mediating the contractile response to neurokinin agonists in the guinea-pig trachea. Regulatory Peptides, 22, 93.

Ireland, S.J., Hagan, R.M., Bailey, F, Jordan, C.C. and Stephens-Smiths, M.L. (1990). Receptors mediating neurokinin-induced contraction of the guinea-pig isolated trachea. Br. J. Pharmacol., 99, 63P.

Maggi, C.A., Patachinni, R., Rovero, P. and Meli, A. (1989). The hamster isolated trachea: a new preparation for studying NK_2-receptors. Eur. J. Pharmacol., 166, 435-440.

AAS 31:
Mediators in
Airway Hyperreactivity

INHIBITION BY CALCITONIN GENE-RELATED PEPTIDE OF AGONIST-INDUCED BRONCHOCONSTRICTION IN VARIOUS MAMMALS INCLUDING MAN

A. Cadieux and C. Lanoue

Department of Pharmacology, Faculty of Medicine, University of Sherbrooke, Sherbrooke, Quebec, Canada J1H 5N4

SUMMARY: The effect of calcitonin gene-related peptide (CGRP) on the smooth muscle of mammalian airways has been investigated in vitro. CGRP itself lacked contractile activity but reduced responses evoked by bronchoconstrictor agents via a post-junctionnal action. The inhibitory effect of CGRP was concentration-related and greatest in distal airways. The results suggest that CGRP may contribute to regulating muscular tone in the tracheobronchial tree.

INTRODUCTION

Calcitonin gene-related peptide (CGRP) is a 37 amino acid peptide which is localised to sensory nerves in the lung of several species including human (Cadieux et al. 1986; Martling & al. 1988). Its vasodilatory action on pulmonary vessels has been well documented but its involvement in the control of the airway smooth muscle tone remains unknown (McCormack & al. 1988; Martling & al. 1988). Accordingly, in the present study, we have investigated the functionnal effects of CGRP on airway smooth muscle preparations obtained from various levels of the respiratory tract.

MATERIALS AND METHODS

Male Sprague Dawley rats (200-250 g) and Hartley albino male guinea pigs (300-400 g) were used. Tracheal chains, bronchial and parenchymal strips (approximately 15 mm X 3 mm X 3 mm) were prepared. Human small bronchi (2-4 mm, i.d.) were dissected out from macroscopically normal lung specimens obtained 4-8 h post mortem and cut into spirals. Finally, bronchial and parenchymal strips were collected from actively sensitized guinea pig to ovalbumin. Sensitization was performed by injecting 100 mg i.p. and 100 mg s.c. on day 1 and a further 10 mg i.p. on day 8. Animals were killed 2 weeks later. Each tissue preparation was set up for isometric recording (Grass Instruments) in a 5 ml organ bath (oxygenated Krebs solution, pH 7.4, 37°C) under a resting tension of 1 g. After 60 min of equilibration, the following experiments were carried out on the preparations: (1) The effect of CGRP on the muscle tone. (2) The ability of CGRP to influence the contraction elicited by single concentration of various well known bronchoconstrictor agents and (3) The effect of tetrodotoxin (TTX), propranolol or indomethacin on the action of CGRP.

All data are given as mean values $\pm$ s.e.m. Student's t-test for unpaired data was used to evaluate the differences in the means.

RESULTS

CGRP (10^{-10} to 10^{-6}M) lacked contractile activity on all airway preparations. However, when added 2 min before some agonist standards, CGRP concentration-dependently reduced the responses elicited by the spasmogens in most preparations tested (Fig. 1). In rat airways CGRP antagonized the bronchoconstrictor effect of 5-HT (5 X 10^{-7}M); the inhibitory action of the peptide being more powerfully expressed in parenchymal strips than in trachea. At a concentration of 10^{-6}M, CGRP reached an inhibitory effect of 42.6 ± 3.8% in lung parenchyma ($p<0.05$), 31.3 ± 3.8% in main bronchus ($p<0.05$) and 13.4 ± 0.65% in trachea ($p>0.05$) (Fig. 1A). Similar results were obtained with carbamylcholine (10^{-7}M) as the spasmogen with the exception of a higher reduction (63.3 ± 5.9%, $p<0.05$) in the agonist-induced response in parenchymal strips (not shown). Propranolol, indomethacin or TTX (each 10^{-6}M) did not alter the inhibitory effect of CGRP in these preparations. In human bronchus, the maximal decrease in the contraction evoked by 10^{-6}M carbachol following the administration of 10^{-6}M CGRP amounted to 78.7 ± 7% ($p<0.05$) (Fig. 1B). In airways from untreated guinea pig, CGRP (10^{-6}M) reduced the excitatory effect of SP (5 X 10^{-8}M) by 20 ± 1.5% in main bronchus ($p<0.05$) and by 47 ± 3% in parenchymal strips ($p<0.05$) of the controls, respectively (Fig. 1C). In contrast, the maximal reduction of SP-evoked contraction by CGRP (10^{-6}M) in similar preparations obtained from sensitized guinea pig were much lower and averaged 17.7 ± 10% ($p<0.05$) in parenchyma and less than 5% ($p<0.05$) in main bronchus.

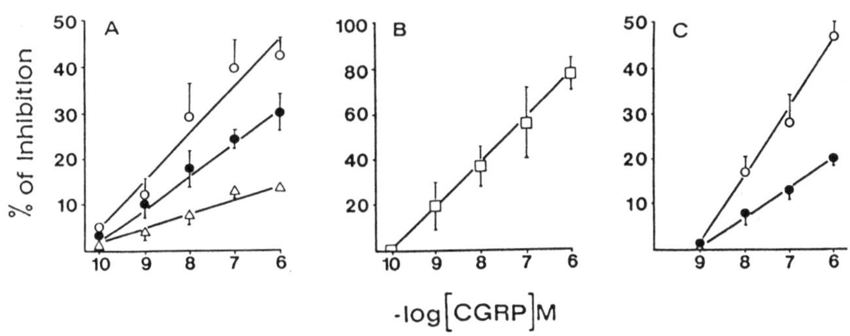

Figure 1: Concentration-dependent inhibition of responses to (A) 5-HT (5 X 10^{-7}M), (B) carbamylcholine (10^{-6}M) and (C) substance P (5 X 10^{-8}M) by CGRP in (A) rat, (B) human and (C) guinea pig isolated airways. The values (means ± s.e.m.) are expressed as percent of controls (n= 3 to 10). (○) parenchyma, (●) bronchus, (△) trachea and (□) human bronchus (2-4 mm i.d.).

DISCUSSION

The present study shows that CGRP, itself, is without contractile effect but has a marked ability to suppress in a concentration-related manner, contractions induced by other agents in rat, guinea pig and human isolated airways. Pharmacological analysis has revealed that the inhibition is presumably direct and that the receptors are located on smooth muscle cells. Interestingly, the inhibitory effect of CGRP was apparent in nanomolar concentrations and was more marked in parenchymal strips than in trachea. This would be in keeping with the demonstration of receptors with high affinity for CGRP in distal airways (Mak and Barnes, 1988). CGRP may therefore be of functionnal importance mainly in the periphery of the tracheobronchial tree. Finally, the decrease in the responsiveness of the airways from sensitized guinea pig to the anti-bronchoconstrictor action of CGRP suggests that the functional effect of CGRP may be altered in some pathophysiological states.

ACKNOWLEDGEMENTS: This work was supported by the Fonds de la Recherche en Santé du Québec (F.R.S.Q.)

REFERENCES

Cadieux, A., Springall, D.R., Mulderry, P.K., Rodrigo, J., Ghatei, M.A., Terenghi, G., Bloom, S.R. and Polak, J.M. (1986). Occurence, distribution and ontogeny of CGRP immunoreactivity in the rat lower respiratory tract: effect of capsaicin treatment and surgical denervations. Neuroscience 19: 605-627.

Mak, J.C.W. and Barnes, P.J. (1988). Autoradiographic localization of calcitonin gene-related peptide (CGRP) binding sites in human and guinea pig lung. Peptides 9: 957-963.

Martling, C.R., Saria, A., Fischer, J.A., Hockfelt, T. and Lundberg, J.M. (1988). Calcitonin gene-related peptide and the lung; neuronal co-existence with substance P, release by capsaicin and vasodilatory effects. Regul. Pept. 20, 125-139.

McCormack, D.G., Mak, J.C.W. and Barnes, P.J. (1988). Calcitonin gene-related peptide (CGRP) causes non-endothelial dependent relaxation of human pulmonary arteries and veins. Am. Rev. Respir. Dis. 137, 372 (abstract).

AAS 31:
Mediators in
Airway Hyperreactivity

SENSORY NEUROPEPTIDES ARE INVOLVED IN CIGARETTE SMOKE INDUCED AIRWAY HYPERREACTIVITY IN GUINEA-PIG

L. Daffonchio, A. Hernandez and *C. Omini

Institute of Pharmacological Sciences, University of Milan, Italy and *Research & Development Laboratories, Dompé Farmaceutici S.p.A., Milan, Italy

SUMMARY: Acute cigarette smoke exposure in anaesthetized guinea-pigs resulted in non-specific airway hyperreactivity associated with inflammatory cell influx within the lung. Sensory neuropeptides seem to be involved in the genesis of smoke induced airway hyperreactivity.

INTRODUCTION

Cigarette smoke is a well known agent responsible for several pathological alteration. Within the respiratory system, increased airway resistance, smooth muscle hypertrophy, globet cell hyperplasia and inflammation have been described after smoke exposure (US Public Health Service, 1984). Moreover, increased airway reactivity to different stimuli has been reported in smokers (Buczko et al., 1984; Mullen et al., 1986).

In the present study we investigated the occurence of airway hyperreactivity induced in anaesthetized guinea-pigs by direct cigarette smoke exposure, and the possible link of this phenomenon with the development of lung inflammation. Moreover, we verified the possible role of different mediators in the genesis of smoke induced airway hyperreactivity.

MATERIALS AND METHODS

Smoke induced airway hyperreactivity: Male Dunkin-Hartley guinea-pigs (450-550 g; Rodentia, Italy) were anaesthetized with urethane (1.2 g/kg i.p.), tracheostomized and artificially ventilated (50 strokes/min with 5 ml air; Rodent Ventilator, Basile, Italy).

Pulmonary inflation pressure (PIP, mmHg) was recorded through a pressure transducer (Bentley Trantec 800) connected to the ventilation circuit, on a Basile 7051 pen recorder.

The smoke was generated by a high tar commercially available cigarette directly connected to the ventilation circuit. Animals inhaled the smoke for 10 s/min for 10 min.

The development of airway hyperreactivity was assessed as the increase in the bronchoconstriction induced by a single dose of acetylcholine (Ach, ranging from 10 to 30 μg/kg i.v.) tested before and at different times after smoke exposure. In some experiments, dose-response curves for histamine (Hist, 3-100 μg/kg i.v.) were obtained 5 min after smoke inhalation and at the same time interval after initial stabilization in control animals.

Bronchoalveolar lavage: The bronchoalveolar lavage (BAL) was performed 5 and 50 min after smoke delivery in separate animals. The lung cavity was gently washed through the trachea with 10 x 3 ml of saline (37°C). BAL fluid was centrifuged for 10 min at 800 g and the pellet resuspended in phosphate buffered saline for total and differential cell count determination, as previously described (Hernandez et al., 1988).

Pharmacological treatments: Capsaicin desensitization was obtained following the modified method of Gamse et al. (1981). Hydrocortisone was administered at the dose of 50 mg/Kg s.c. 24 and 2 h before smoke exposure.
In some animals both cervical vagi were cut at the beginning of the experiments.

RESULTS

Acute cigarette smoke inhalation in anaesthetized guinea-pig resulted in the development of airway hyperreactivity. As shown in Figure 1, the bronchoconstriction induced by Ach (17.7±2.7

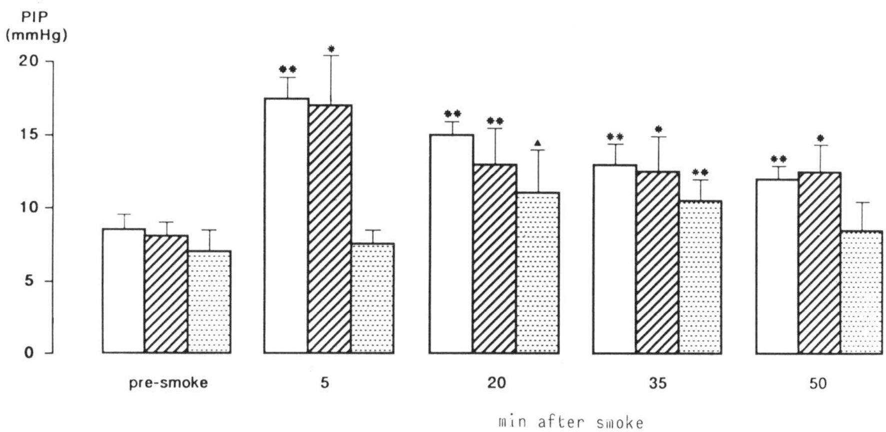

Fig. 1. Effect of cigarette smoke exposure on the bronchoconstriction induced by acetylcholine in normal (blank box, n=16), vagotomized (right diagonal, n=6) and capsaicin desensitized (filled box, n=7) anaesthetized guinea-pigs. Data are expressed as increase in pulmonary inflation pressure (PIP) over the basal values and represent the mean±SE of n° experiments.
*$p < 0.05$, **$p < 0{,}01$, as compared to pre-smoke values (paired Student's t test).
▲ $p < 0.01$, as compared to normal at the same time (one way Dunnett's test).

µg/Kg i.v.; n=16) was significantly ($p<0.01$) increased up to 50 min after smoke exposure when compared to pre-smoke value. Cervical vagotomy did not modify the degree and the time-course of smoke induced hyperreactive phenomenon. On the other hand, depletion of sensory neuropeptides due to capsaicin desensitization almost completely inhibited the development of smoke induced airway hyperreactivity (Fig. 1).

In these animals, the bronchoconstrictions induced by Ach (24.3±4.3 µg/Kg i.v.; n=7) before and 5 min after smoke exposure were comparable. Ach effect was slightly even significantly ($p<0.01$) potentiated only at 35 min after cigarette smoke inhalation.

Airway hyperreactivity, triggered by acute cigarette smoke exposure, was paralleled by an influx of inflammatory cells into the lung. Total cell number recovered in BAL fluid 5 and 50 min after smoke inhalation was significantly ($p<0.01$) enhanced when compared to controls (Table 1).

Table 1. Effect of active cigarette smoke exposure on proinflammatory cell count in guinea-pig BAL fluid

	Control	5 min	50 min
Total cells	9.84±0.71	15.05±0.82*	14.17±1.60*
Neutrophils	0.34±0.18	0.43±0.32	0.74±0.24
Eosinophils	0.20±0.04	0.67±0.15*	0.36±0.15
Macrophages	8.77±0.47	13.35±0.66**	12.49±1.30*

Data are expressed as cells x 10^6/30 ml BAL fluid and represent the mean±SEM of 4 experiments. BAL was performed in control animals and 5 and 50 min after smoke exposure in separate guinea-pigs.

*$p<0.05$, **$p<0.01$, as compared to controls (one way Dunnett's test).

Within the different classes of cells, the number of eosinophils was markedly and significantly ($p < 0.05$) increased 5 min after smoke delivery. An increased number of macrophages was observed 5 and 50 min after smoke exposure.

Histamine dose-response curves (Figure 2), obtained in smoke exposed animals (n=9), were also significantly ($p < 0.01$) shifted to the left of those obtained in control animals (n=11), with a DR of 1.8 (95% conf. lim. 1.3-2.5). In animals treated with hydrocortisone, smoke exposure significantly ($p < 0.05$) shifted to the left of controls Histamine dose-response curves (n=6 for each group; DR=1.7, 95% conf. lim. 1.0-2.8).

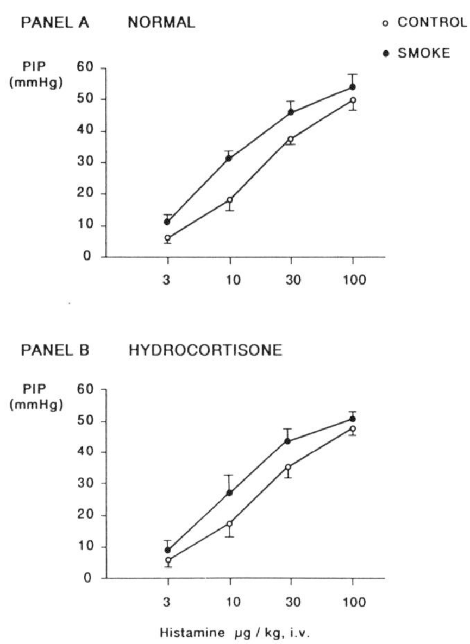

Fig. 2. Effects of cigarette smoke exposure on the bronchoconstriction induced by histamine (Hist) in normal (panel A) and hydrocortisone (panel B) anaesthetized guinea-pigs. Hist dose-response curves were obtained in control (open circle) and smoke exposed (filled circles) animals. Data are expressed as increase in pulmonary inflation pressure (PIP) over the basal values and represent the mean±SE of at least 6 experiments.

DISCUSSION

The present results clearly demonstrate the occurrence of non-specific airway hyperreactivity after acute cigarette smoke exposure in anaesthetized guinea-pig. This phenomenon was rapid in onset, being evident 5 min after smoke inhalation, and lasted up to 50 min.

A wide range of mediators has been demonstrated to play a role in the genesis of airway hyperreactivity in different experimental conditions (Boushey et al. 1980). As far as the smoke induced airway hyperresponsiveness is concerned, our data suggest that the cholinergic reflex does not partecipate to this phenomenon, since in vagotomized animals no difference was observed either in the degree and time course of airway hyperreactivity. A possible role of Ach, released from vagal nerves, in the increased effectiveness of Hist, seen after smoke exposure, has been reported (Hulbert et al. 1985). However, our data, together with that published by Lunberg et al., demonstrating the inability of hexamethonium to prevent smoke induced tracheal extravasation, indicate a marginal role for the cholinergic mechanism. On the other hand, our data support the involvement of sensory neuropeptides in the genesis of smoke induced airway hyperreactivity, since their depletion due to capsaicin desensitization almost completely abolished the capacity of cigarette smoke to potentiate Ach response. These results are in line with evidences for a role of sensory neuropeptides in smoke induced bronchoconstriction (Lunberg et al. 1982) and airway oedema (Lundberg et al. 1983). In addition, Omini et al. (1989) demonstrated the capacity of exogenously administered substance P to potentiate Ach induced bronchoconstriction in guinea-pigs. On the other hand the present results do not support the role of arachidonic acid metabolites in smoke induced hyperresponsiveness, since the pretreatment with hydrocortisone, did not modify the capacity of cigarette smoke to potentiate Hist induced bronchoconstriction.

As far as other pathological alterations are concerned, migration of inflammatory cells into the airway lumen has been observed in parallel with the development of smoke induced increase in airway responsiveness; these data support a link also between airway hyperreactivity induced by smoke and an inflammatory reaction (O'Byrne et al. 1986).

Eosinophil number was particularly increased after smoke exposure; however, the fact that the number of these cells returned to control values within 50 min whereas the hyperreactivity, lasted up to this time, indicates that an interaction with other cells and mediators is needed to maintain the hyperreactive phenomenon during the time. Macrophages might be a good candidate in fact, these cells have been indeed indicated to play a role also in other respiratory alterations induced by cigarette smoke (Chang et al. 1986).

REFERENCES

US Public Health Service, Washington, DC, Government Printing Office (1984) DHHS (PHS) 84-50205

Buczko, G.B., Day, A., Vanderdoelen, J.L., Boucher, R., Zamel. N. (1984) Am. Rev. Respir. Dis. 129, 12-14.

Mullen, J.B.R., Wiggs, B.R., Wright, J.L., Hogg, J.C., Pare' P.D.(1986) Am. Rev. Respir. Dis. 133, 120-125.

Hernandez, A., Daffonchio, L., Brunelli, G., Pasargiklian, R., Omini, C. (1988), Pharmac. Res. Comm. 20, 983-992.

Gamse, R., Wax, A., Zigmond, R.E., Leeman, S.A. (1981), Neuroscience, 6, 437-441.
Bausbey, H.A., Holtzman, M.J., Sheller, J.R., Nadel, J.A. (1980), Am. Rev. Respir. Dis., 121, 389-413.
Hulbert, W.M.N. McLean, T., Hogg, J.C. (1985) Am. Rev. Respir. Dis., 132, 7-11.
Lundberg, J.M., Martling, C.R., Saria, A., Folkers, K., Rosell, S. (1983), Neuroscience, 10, 1361-1368.
Lundberg, J.M., Saria, A. (1982), Acta Physiol. Scand., 116, 477-480.
Omini, C., Brunelli, G., Hernandez, A., Daffonchio, L. (1989) Eur. J. Pharmacol., 163, 195-197
Chang, J.C., Lesser, M., Yoo, O.H., Orlowski, M. (1986) Am. Rev. Respir. Dis., 134, 538-541.
O'Byrne, P.M. (1986) Chest, 90, 575-577

AAS 31:
Mediators in
Airway Hyperreactivity

AMINO ACIDS AS MODULATORS OF CHOLINERGIC NERVES IN AIRWAYS

Pål Aas and Frode Fonnum

Norwegian Defence Research Establishment, Division for Environmental Toxicology, P.O. Box 25, N-2007 Kjeller, Norway.

SUMMARY: The bronchial smooth muscle of rat was examined for contractile responses to excitatory amino acids. The electrical field stimulation (EFS) which induces release of ACh, induced contraction which was enhanced by exogenous L-glutamate (L-glu). The ED_{50} of L-glu was 3.5 ± 0.1 mM. Inhibition of the release by TTX or by HC-3 completely abolished the potentiation of the EFS-induced contraction by L-glu. The effect of L-glu is therefore probably a prejunctional effect. Concentrations of L-glu higher than 22 mM inhibited the EFS evoked contractions, and enhanced the tonus of the muscle by a postjunctional stimulation. The ED_{50} of ACh was not altered by L-glu. In contrast, an increase of the intrinsic activity (α) of ACh was seen, providing evidence for a postjunctional potentiation of ACh induced contraction. L-glu did not inhibit AChE-activity at concentrations up to 50 mM, indicating that the effect is not due to an accumulation of ACh. A relaxation of the EFS-induced bronchial smooth muscle contraction was seen with high concentrations of D-glu, L-asp, L-α - amino adipate and ibotenate. Neither L-GDEE nor DL-APV had any inhibitory effect on L-glu and L-asp induced alteration of EFS-evoked contraction or on the L-glu enhanced tonus of the bronchial smooth muscle. Kainate, NMDA and quisqualate had only minor transient potentiating effects on the EFS-induced contraction. The results provide evidence for an apparent new L-glu receptor in rat bronchi with different specificity for glutamate agonists and antagonists than the L-glu receptor described in the CNS and the receptor seems to be located prejunctionally to enhance release of ACh. The response to L-glu might explain some of the peripheral symtoms described as the "Chinese Restaurant Syndrome".

The amino acids glutamate and aspartate function as important excitatory neurotransmitters in the mammalian central nervous system (CNS) (Curtis et al., 1960; Fonnum, 1984) and in invertebrate striated muscle (Usherwood, 1981; Crawford and McBurney, 1986). Three subtypes of receptors for acidic amio acids have been described based on the selectivity of specific agonist, namely the NMDA (N-methyl-D-aspartate), quisqualate and kainate receptors. Ibotenate is an agonist for the NMDA receptor but is also a weak agonist for the quisqualate receptor (for review, see Foster and Fagg, 1984).

In vertebrates, peripheral receptors for excitatory amino acids have been described in amphibians (Nistri and Costani, 1979). In mammals, however, specific actions for excitatory amino acids in the peripheral nervous system have not yet been established. A recent report provides evidence for a contractile effect of L-glu and L-asp in the guinea-pig ileum (Moroni et al., 1986). Their results indicate that a NMDA type receptor exists in the myenteric plexus. We provide evidence for the specific excitatory amino acid modulation (by L-glu) of smooth muscle contraction in the respiratory organ and show that the receptor involved is different from the NMDA receptor in the guinea-pig gut.

MATERIALS AND METHODS

Broncial smooth muscle from the albino rat was isolated and mounted in an organ bath for measurement of contraction (Aas and Helle, 1982). The Krebs buffer (37°C, pH = 7.4) had the following composition (mM): NaCl, 118.4; KCl, 4.7; $CaCl_2$, 2.6; $MgSO_4$, 1.2; $NaHCO_3$, 24.9; KH_2PO_4, 1.2; Glucose, 11.1. The buffer was gassed with 95% O_2 and 5% CO_2. For EFS the bronchi were mounted between platinum electrodes and stimulated (20 Hz, 1.0 ms, supramaximal voltage) by a Grass Stimulator. The preparations were given a preload of 1.0 g and equilibrated for 60 min before start of the experiments. The contractions were recorded isometrically by Grass Force Displacement Transducers (FT-03C) and monitored on a Grass Polygraph (Model 7) fitted with amplifiers (7 P 1A). For determination of acetylcholinesterase (AChE) activity the rat bronchi were homogenized (10% w/v) in 20 mM sodium-potassium phosphate buffer (pH 7.4) (glass/glass homogeniser, 20 strokes, 720 r.p.m., ice-cold). The AChE activity was determined at 30°C by the radiochemical method of Sterri and Fonnum (1978) in the presence and absence of L-glu).

The means and standard error of the mean (S.E.M) were calculated for all data. Statistical analyses were done with Student's t-test (two-tailed).

RESULTS

Previously, electrical stimulation has shown to induce release of ACh from the cholinergic nerves in the airways (Aas and Helle, 1982; Aas and Fonnum, 1986). L-glutamate (L-glu) specifically enhanced the electrical evoked contraction of bronchial smooth muscle (Fig. 1). The maximal increase in contraction by L-glu was 104%. The concentration of L-glu that induced a half-maximal response (ED_{50}) was 3.5 ± 0.1 mM (n=30). Higher concentrations (> 22 mM), however, inhibited the electrical-field induced contractions. L-glu, in concentrations having presynaptic activity (< 22 mM), had no effect on the contraction induced by exogenous ACh. The concentration of ACh inducing half-maximal contraction (ED_{50}) and the intrinsic activity (α) of ACh were not

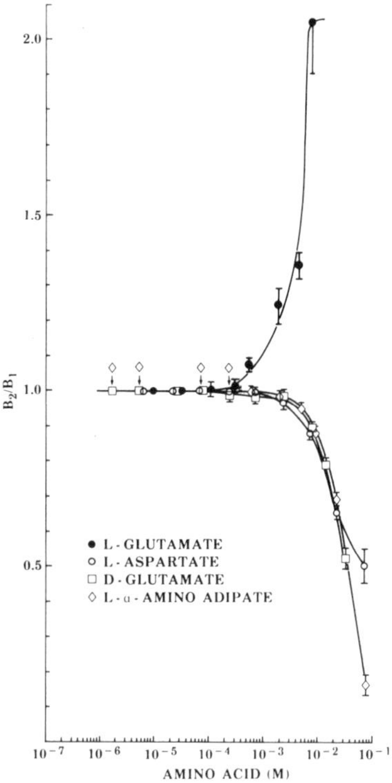

Figure 1. The effect of L-glutamate, D-glutamate, L-aspartate and L-α-amino adipate on prejunctional transmural stimulation of the parasympathetic nerves in rat bronchial smooth muscle. The prejunctional effect is shown as an increase or decrease in the ratio B_2/B_1 where B_2 is the response after exposure to the amino acid. Results are expressed as the mean result ±SEM of 23, 10, 4 and 3 experiments respectively.

changed (Table I). Atropine (1.1 μM) reduced the presynaptic effect of L-glu by 32% (n = 7). The effect of L-glu was not a result of enhanced levels of ACh due to inhibition of the acetylcholinesterase activity (not shown). D-glutamate (D-glu), L-aspartate (L-asp) and L-α-amino adipate (L-α-aa), however, reduced the electrical induced contraction (Fig. 1). The reduction of contraction was 50% at 31 mM of D-glu. Neither of the antagonists L-glutamic acid diethyl ester (L-GDEE) (1.0 mM, n = 6) and 2-amino-5-phosphonovalerate (DL-APV) (20 μM and 1.0 mM, n = 6) had any effects on L-glu enhanced or L-asp reduced electrical field induced contraction. The apparent affinity (ED_{50}) and intrinsic activity (α) of L-glu was not changed (not shown). NMDA, kainate and quisqualate had no effects on the bronchial smooth muscle or on the electrical induced contractions in concentrations up to 1–10 mM (not shown).

Table I. Apparent affinity (ED_{50}) and intrinsic activity (α) of ACh in the absence and presence of L-glutamate (L-glu)

	ED_{50} (μM)	α
Control	63 ± 35	1.00
L-glu (8.6 mM)	69 ± 35 ns	1.12 ± 0.08 ns
L-glu (62.0 mM)	85 ± 42 ns	1.21 ± 0.08 *

The results are expressed as the mean ± SEM of 6 experiments.
$^{*}p < 0.05$; $^{ns}p > 0.05$.

DISCUSSION

The presently described results provide evidence for a specific effect of L-glu on peripheral cholinergic nerves. Although receptors for excitatory amino acids have been proposed to exist in the guinea-pig myenteric plexus (Moroni *et al.*, 1986), these receptors are of the NMDA type and not specific for L-glu, as was seen in rat bronchial smooth muscle. The bronchial L-glu receptor was not antagonized by the NMDA antagonist APV or the quisqualate receptor antagonist GDEE, which provide evidence for the receptor to be different from the NMDA receptor in the guinea-pig.

The stereoselectivity of the L-glu receptor was shown by the fact that only L-glu, and not the stereoisomer D-glu, potentiated the electrical field induced contractions. Such a specificity has previously not been described for the L-glu receptor. Furthermore, L-aspartate and L-α-aa, which gave the opposite effect to L-glu and reduced the contraction induced by endogenously released ACh, provided further evidence for a specific excitatory receptor for L-glu. The prejunctional location of this receptor was shown in experiments in which L-glu had no effect on the application of exogenous ACh.

The possible involvement of this receptor in the "Chinese Restaurant Syndrome" is of particular interest, since the dose of glutamate that causes asthmatic symptoms in humans, 1.5 – 12 g per os (Schaumburg *et al.*, 1969) corresponds to a systemic concentration of 0.1 – 1.0 mM glutamate. This is close to the concentrations of L-glu that caused contraction in our experiments. Furthermore, Schaumburg reported that it was only the L-form that induced symptoms in their subjects, which is also in agreement with the present experiments. Ghadimi and colleagues (1971 and 1972) suggested that the symptoms show some resemblance to parasympathomimetic effects, and showed that the symptoms were attenuated by atropine and enhanced by the acetylcholinesterase inhibitor prostigmine. These effects could well be explained by the periopherally located prejunctional glutamate receptors described in this paper.

REFERENCES

Aas, P., and Fonnum, F. (1986), Acta. Physiol. Scand. 127, 335–342.
Aas, P., and Helle, K.B. (1982), Neurotensin receptors in the rat bronchi, Regul. Pept. 3, 405–413.
Crawford, A.C., and McBurney, R.N. (1976), The post-synaptic action of some putative excitatory transmitter substances, Proc. R. Soc. Lodon B 192, 481–489.
Curtis, D.R., Phillis, J.W., and Watkins, J.C. (1960), The chemical exitation of spinal neurons by certain acidic amino acids, J. Physiol. 150, 656–682.
Fonnum, F. (1984), Glutamate: A neurotransmitter in the mammalian brain, J. Neurochem.42, I–II.
Foster, A.C., and Fagg, G.E. (1984), Acidic amino acid binding sites in mammalian neuronal membranes: Their characteristics and relationship to synaptic receptors, Brain Res. R7, 103–164.
Ghadimi, H., and Kumar, S. (1972), Current status of monosodium glutamate, Am. J. Clin. Nutr. 25, 643–646.
Ghadimi, H., Kumar, S., and Abaci, F. (1971), Studies on monosodium glutamate ingestion. 1. Biochemical explanation of Chinese restaurant syndrome, Biochem. Med. 5, 447–56.
Moroni, F., Luzzi, S., Franchi-Micheli, S., and Zilletti, L. (1986), The presence of N-methyl-D-aspartate-type receptors for glutamic acid in the guinea-pig myenteric plexus, Neurosci. Lett. 68, 57–62.
Nistri, A., and Costanti, A. (1979), Pharmacological characterization of different types of GABA and glutamate receptors in vertebrates and invertebrates, Progr. Neurobiol. 13, 117–235.
Schaumburg, H.H., Byck, R., Gerstl, B.R., and Mashman, J.H. (1969), Monosodium L-glutamate: Its pharmacology and role in the Chinese restaurant syndrome, Science 163, 826–828.
Sterri, S.H., and Fonnum, F. (1978), Isolation of organic anions by extraction with liquid anion exchangers and its application to micromethods for acetylcholinesterase and 4-aminobutyrate aminotransferase, European J. Biochem. 91, 215–222.
Usherwood, P.N.R. (1981), Glutamate synapse and receptors in insect muscle, In: Glutamate as a neurotransmitter, Eds. G. Di-Chiara and G.L. Gessal (Raven Press, New York), p. 183–192.

AAS 31:
Mediators in
Airway Hyperreactivity

CONTRACTILE EFFECTS AND RECEPTOR DISTRIBUTIONS FOR ENDOTHELIN-1 (ET-1) IN HUMAN AND ANIMAL AIRWAYS

R.G. Goldie, P.J. Henry, J.W. Paterson, J.M.H. Preuss and P.J. Rigby

Department of Pharmacology, University of Western Australia, Perth, Nedlands, 6009, Australia

SUMMARY: ET-1 caused concentration-dependent, sustained contraction of all airway preparations tested and was most potent in mouse trachea, with rat trachea, human bronchus and guinea-pig trachea approximately 5, 10 and 70 fold less sensitive respectively. Human non-asthmatic and asthmatic bronchi were approximately equi-sensitive to ET-1. Quantitative light microscopic autoradiography demonstrated high levels of specific [^{125}I]-ET-1 binding sites in airway smooth muscle of rat trachea > human asthmatic bronchus = human non-asthmatic bronchus > mouse trachea >> guinea-pig trachea. High levels of specific ET-1 binding were also revealed in peripheral airways and in alveolar wall tissue in human, rat and mouse lung. In a limited sample of asthmatic airway smooth muscle ET-1 receptor function and density was not elevated.

INTRODUCTION

ET-1 is a potent vasoconstrictor peptide released by the vascular endothelium under hypoxic conditions (Yanagisawa et al., 1988). This peptide may play a role in asthma, a disease involving airway hypoxia, since it is synthesized in the airway epithelium (McCumber et al., 1989; Rozengurt et al., 1990) and causes sustained elevations of airway smooth muscle tone (Maggi et al., 1989; Henry et al., 1990). ET-1 has also been reported to be a powerful mitogen of vascular smooth muscle (Hirata et al., 1989) and may be responsible for the airway smooth muscle hyperplasia sometimes reported in human asthma (Dunnill, 1971). The present study examines the contractile potency of ET-1 and the distribution of specific binding sites for this peptide in the lung of various species, including man.

METHODS

Organ bath studies: Isolated airway ring preparations were suspended in organ baths containing 3 ml of Krebs-bicarbonate solution at 37°C, bubbled with 5% CO_2 in O_2. Changes in isometric tension in airway smooth muscle in response to cumulative concentrations of ET-1 (0.1 nM - 0.3μM) were recorded via FT03C force-displacement transducers (Grass Instruments).

Quantitative autoradiography: Slide-mounted frozen sections of animal and human (non-asthmatic n = 3 lung samples; asthmatic n = 3 lung samples) central and peripheral airway tissues were incubated with ^{125}I-ET-1 (0.1 - 2 nM) for 60 min at 22°C in buffer (50 mM Tris-HCl, 100 mM NaCl, 0.25% BSA, pH 7.4). Non-specific binding was assessed in the presence of 1 μM ET-1. Tissue sections were washed to remove unbound ligand and buffer salts, dried under a stream of cold dry air and opposed to nuclear track emulsion-coated (NTB-2) coverslips. These assemblies were placed in light-tight x-ray cassettes for 6 days and autoradiograms produced. Specific grain densities were then determined over selected tissue types as described by Henry et al. (1990).

RESULTS

Organ bath studies: ET-1 caused concentration-dependent contraction of all central airway preparations tested and was most potent in mouse trachea > rat trachea > human non-asthmatic bronchus = human asthmatic bronchus > guinea-pig trachea. Guinea-pig trachea was also the least responsive to ET-1, producing only 32% of the maximal response to carbachol at the highest concentration used (i.e. 0.3 μM). EC_{30} values are presented in Table I. In contrast, EC_{50} values for carbachol varied by less than 3-fold between these species.

Table I : Spasmogenic potency of ET-I in airway smooth muscle

	*EC_{30} (nM)	95% confidence limits	n
Mouse trachea	3.4	2.4 - 5.0	11
Rat trachea	16.8	11.2 - 25.2	6
Guinea-pig trachea	241.0	126.0 - 462.0	
Human bronchus			
non-asthmatic	35.2	5.4 - 231.0	3
asthmatic	53.0	-	1

*Data reproduced from Henry et al. (1990) Br. J. Pharmacol (in press)

Quantitative autoradiography: Light microscopic autoradiography revealed high densities of specific ^{125}I-ET-1 binding sites in tracheal airway smooth muscle in the rat > mouse >> guinea-pig. High levels of specific binding were also evident in both non-asthmatic and asthmatic human bronchial smooth muscle, alveolar wall tissue and in peripheral blood vessels. Specific binding in airway smooth muscle was saturable, with dissociation constants (Kd) in the range 0.11-0.43 nM (Henry et al., 1990).

DISCUSSION

ET-1 produced sustained contraction of human and animal isolated airway smooth muscle preparations. In human bronchus, ET-1 was about three times more potent than carbachol. High densities of specific ^{125}I-ET-1 binding sites were localized to airway smooth muscle, some of which presumably mediate contractile responses. High levels of specific binding were also associated with alveolar wall tissue, although the cell types and the role of these sites is not known. Asthma does not appear to involve increased ET-1 binding site density or increased receptor sensitivity in bronchial airway smooth muscle.

Acknowledgement: This research was supported by the National Health and Medical Research Council of Australia.

REFERENCES

Dunnill, M.S. (1971) Pathology of Asthma. In: Identification of Asthma. (R. Porter and J. Birch, Eds.) Churchill, Livingstone, London: pp. 35-40.

Henry, P.J., Rigby, P.J., Self, G.J., Preuss, J.M.H. and Goldie, R.G. (1990) Relationship between endothelin-1 binding site densities and constrictor activities in human and animal airway smooth muscle. Br. J. Pharmacol. (in press).

Hirata, Y., Takagi, Y., Fukuda, Y. and Marumo, F. (1989) Endothelin is a potent mitogen in rat vascular smooth muscle cells. Atherosclerosis, 78, 225-228.

Maggi, C.A., Patacchini, R., Giulani, S. and Meli, A. (1989) Potent contractile effect of endothelin in isolated guinea-pig airways. Eur. J. Pharmacol., 160, 179-182.

MacCumber, M.W., Ross, C.A., Glaser, B.M. and Snyder, S.H. (1989). Endothelin: Visualization of mRNAs by *in situ* hybridization provides evidence for local action. Proc. Natl. Acad. Sci. USA., 86, 7285-7289.

Rozengurt, N., Springall, D. R. and Polak, J. M. (1990) Localization of endothelin-like immunoreactivity in airway epithelium of rats and mice. J. Pathol., 160, 5-8.

Yanagisawa, M., Kurihara, H., Kimura, S., Tomoke, Y., Kobayashi, M., Mitsui, Y., Yazaki, Y., Goto, K. and Mazaki, T. (1988) A novel potent vasoconstrictor peptide produced by vascular endothelial cells. Nature, 332, 411-415.

AAS 31:
Mediators in
Airway Hyperreactivity

BINDING CHARACTERISTICS OF [^{125}I]ENDOTHELIN-1 IN GUINEA-PIG TRACHEA AND ITS DISPLACEMENT BY ENDOTHELIN-1, ENDOTHELIN-3 AND ENDOTHELIN (16-21).

E.J. Tschirhart, J.T. Pelton and C.R. Jones.

Merrell Dow Research Institute, 16 rue d'Ankara, 67084 Strasbourg Cedex, France.

SUMMARY: The presence of binding sites for endothelin-1 (ET-1) and endothelin-3 (ET-3) in airway epithelium, submucosa and smooth muscle of guinea-pig trachea was investigated using *in vitro* autoradiography. We also examined the ability of the C-terminal hexapeptide of endothelin, ET(16-21) to inhibit specific [^{125}I]ET-1 binding. ET-1 appeared to bind to a single class of binding sites (n_H not different from unity). In contrast, n_H values for ET-3 displacement of [^{125}I]ET-1 specific binding were different from unity, suggesting that these peptides bound to more than one site. ET(16-21) did not affect [^{125}I]ET-1 binding. The present results suggest that the binding sites identified in guinea pig airway smooth muscle may be related to receptors mediating contractile responses to the endothelins.

Endothelin-1 (ET-1) induces a contraction of guinea-pig (trachea and bronchus) and human (bronchus) isolated airways (Uchida et al., 1989; Maggi et al., 1989; Tschirhart and Miller, 1990). Recent studies also indicate that endothelin-3 (ET-3) can contract guinea-pig trachea and bronchus (Maggi et al., 1990; Tschirhart and Miller, 1990). Therefore, the presence of binding sites for ET-1 and ET-3 in the airway epithelium, sub-mucosa and smooth muscle of guinea pig trachea was investigated using *in vitro* autoradiography. We also examined the ability of the C-terminal hexapeptide of endothelin, ET(16-21), to inhibit specific [^{125}I]ET-1 binding since this peptide has been suggested to interact with a postulated ET_B receptor in guinea-pig airways (Maggi et al., 1990).

MATERIALS AND METHODS

Tracheas were removed from Dunkin-Hartley guinea-pigs under anaesthesia with pentobarbitone (45 mg/kg). Tracheas were cleaned of connective tissue and frozen on dry ice. Autoradiography was performed on slide-mounted 20 µm serial sections as previously described (Jones et al., 1989). Inhibition studies were performed using varying concentrations of unlabelled ET-1, ET-3 (Peninsula, USA) or ET(16-21)(synthetized at Merrell Dow). Non-specific binding was defined in sections incubated with radiolabelled peptide in the presence of 10 µM unlabelled ET-1. Adjacent slide-mounted sections were stained for histological examination with haematoxylin and eosin. Binding sites on epithelium, sub-mucosa and smooth muscle were quantified as previously described (Jones et al., 1989). Binding and inhibition data were analysed using the computer programs EBDA and LIGAND (Munson and Rodbard, 1980; MacPherson, 1986). In all experiments, results are expressed as means ± s.e.mean of 6 experiments.

RESULTS

Specific binding was 85-95% of total binding. K_d and B_{max} values for ET-1 are indicated in Table I. The greatest density of ET-1 binding sites was observed in the sub-mucosa and the least within the airway epithelium.

Table I: Binding of $[^{125}I]$ET-1 to different regions of guinea-pig trachea.

	K_d (nM)	B_{max} (fmoles/mg prot)
Epithelium	1.41 ± 0.11	44 ± 2
Sub-mucosa	0.88 ± 0.07	693 ± 60
Smooth muscle	2.76 ± 0.21	279 ± 16

Following competition experiments, K_i and n_H values for specific $[^{125}I]$ET-1 binding were determined in the epithelium, sub-mucosa and smooth muscle from guinea-pig trachea. (Table II). ET-1 apparently bound to a single class of binding sites (n_H not different from unity, $P > 0.05$) in all areas studied. In contrast, n_H values for ET-3 displacement of $[^{125}I]$ET-1 specific binding were different from unity ($P < 0.05$). ET(16-21),up to 10^{-5}M, did not significantly inhibit $[^{125}I]$ET-1 binding.

Table II. Inhibition of $[^{125}I]$ET-1 binding by ET-1 and ET-3 in different regions of guinea-pig trachea.

	Endothelin-1		Endothelin-3	
	K_i (nM)	n_H	K_i (nM)	n_H
Epithelium	1.29 ± 0.15	1.11 ± 0.12	12.10 ± 0.39	0.69 ± 0.10
Sub-mucosa	1.34 ± 0.21	0.91 ± 0.08	4.24 ± 0.25	0.75 ± 0.12
Smooth muscle	0.84 ± 0.58	1.05 ± 0.10	2.57 ± 0.47	0.70 ± 0.11

DISCUSSION

These data provide evidence for specific endothelin binding sites within the epithelium, the sub-mucosa and the smooth muscle in guinea-pig trachea. The correlation between the functional activity of ET-1 in guinea-pig trachea *in vitro* (EC_{50} = 3.87 nM) (Tschirhart and Miller, 1990) and its binding constant suggests that the binding sites identified represent functional receptors. Similarly, the lower potency of ET-3 (EC_{50} = 12.96 nM) correlates with its lower binding affinity. The presence of binding sites within the airway epithelium and within the sub-mucosa suggests that endothelins might also regulate other airway functions such as mucus secretion and/or electrolyte movements. Since we have previously shown that the airway epithelium is able to modulate tracheal contractions induced by ET-1 and not by ET-3, these epithelial receptors could be linked to the generation of a relaxant factor (Tschirhart and Miller, 1990). The low Hill coefficients for ET-3 indicate that these peptides interact with more than one binding site in all the regions. Since the C-terminal hexapeptide of endothelin, ET(16-21) is inactive in inhibiting [^{125}I]ET-1 binding, it can be concluded that this peptide does not interact with endothelin receptors in guinea-pig trachea and therefore does not support the concept of receptor classification based on this compound. However, our data do support the existence of multiple endothelin receptor subtypes and the existence of functional endothelin receptors in guinea-pig airways within the sub-mucosa, the smooth muscle and the epithelium.

REFERENCES

Jones, C.R., Hiley, C.R. Pelton, T.J., and Mohr, M.(1989) Autoradiographic vizualization of the binding sites for [^{125}I]endothelin in rat and human brain. Neurosci. Lett., 97, 276-279

Maggi, C.A., Giuliani, S., Patacchini, R., Santicioli, P., Rovero, P., Giachetti, A. and Meli, A.(1989) The C-terminal hexapeptide, endothelin (16-21) discriminates between different endothelin receptors. Eur. J. Pharmacol., 166, 121-122.

Maggi, C.A., Giuliani, S., Santicioli, P., Giachetti, A. and Meli, A.(1990) Further studies on the responses of the guinea-pig isolated bronchus to endothelins and sarafotoxins S6b. Eur. J. Pharmacol., 176, 1-9.

McPherson, G.A.(1986) KINETIC, EBDA, LIGAND and LOWRY: a collection of computer programs for the analysis of radioligand binding experiments, Cambridge, Elsevier.

Munson, P.J. and Rodbard, D.(1980) LIGAND: a versatile computerized approach for the characterization of ligand binding systems. Anal. Biochem., 107, 220-239.

Tschirhart, E. and Miller, R.(1990) Airway epithelium actively metabolises endothelin and modulates endothelin-induced contraction in guinea-pig trachea. Br. J. Pharmacol., 99, 57P.

Uchida, Y., Ninomiya, H., Saotome, M., Nomura, A., Ohtsuka, M., Yanagisawa, M., Goto, K., Masaki, T., and Hasegawa.(1988) Endothelin, a novel vasoconstrictor peptide, as potent bronchoconstrictor. Eur. J. Pharmacol., 154, 227-228.

AAS 31:
Mediators in
Airway Hyperreactivity

ENDOTHELIN-1 INCREASES AIRWAY MUCOSA BLOOD FLOW IN THE PIG

Régis Matran[1-2], Kjell Alving[2], Anette Hemsen[2] and Jan M. Lundberg

[1] Laboratoire d'Explorations Fonctionnelles, Hôpital Cochin 75014 Paris, France. [2] Department of Pharmacology, Karolinska Institut, Box 60400, S-104 01 Stockholm, Sweden.

SUMMARY : The vascular effects of bolus intravenous injections (4.5, 45 and 450 $pmol.kg^{-1}$) of porcine endothelin-1 on the bronchial and nasal circulations were investigated in ten anesthetized pigs. Endothelin-1 produced a dose-dependent and long-lasting increase in bronchial blood flow with a concomitant rise in systemic arterial pressure suggesting vasodilatation. The highest doses of endothelin-1 also caused a slight decrease in the nasal vascular resistance. Furthermore, the vascular responses to endothelin-1 were not modified in systemically capsaicin pretreated animals or after pretreatment with a cyclocoxygenase inhibitor, diclofenac. Our results suggest that endothelin-1 has a potent and regional vasodilator effect of the bronchial circulation.

INTRODUCTION

The endothelial cell releases vasoactive substances in response to various chemical and physical stimuli (Furchgott, 1984 ; Vanhoutte et al., 1988). Endothelin-1 (ET-1), a newly described polypeptide produced by endothelial cells, is a potent vasoconstrictor agent of isolated blood vesels *in vitro*

(Yanagisawa et al., 1988) and of various vascular beds in vivo (Pernow et al., 1989). Furthermore, ET-1 produces regional vasodilatation and decreases systemic blood arterial pressure in the rat (Lippton et al., 1989).
In the present study, we have determined the effects of ET-1 on the airway mucosa blood flow in the pig, in vivo.

MATERIALS AND METHODS

Animal preparations : Eighteen pigs (25-30 kg bwt) were premedicated with ketamine (Parke-Davis, CA, USA ; 20 mg kg^{-1} i.m.), anesthetized with sodium pentobarbitone (ACO ; Stockholm, Sweden ; 20 mg kg^{-1} followed by 3 mg kg^{-1} h^{-1} i.v.)and mechanically ventilated after administration of pancuronium bromide (Organon, The Netherlands ; O.5 mg kg^{-1} i.v.). Catheters were placed into the left femoral artery and vein for recordings of mean arterial blood pressure (MAP) and heart rate and administration of drugs, respectively. Blood flow in the bronchial artery which supplies the tracheobronchial mucosa and the internal maxillary artery which supplies the nasal mucosa were continuously recorded with Transonic flow probes placed around the vessels and connected to an ultrasonic flow meter (T202 S, Transonic System Inc., NY, USA).

Experimental procedure : Increasing doses (4.5, 45 and 450 pmol kg^{-1}) of ET-1 was given intravenously as bolus injections in six control pigs. Between injections, the catheter was thoroughly rinsed. Two days after systemic pretreatment with capsaicin (n = 6) (Fluka Chemie AG, Switzerland) (for details see Matran et al., 1990), ET-1 injections were performed at the same doses to determine whether release of tachykinins was involved in the vascular response. Furthermore, six other pigs were pretreated with a cyclooxygenase inhibitor, diclofenac (Sigma, St Louis, MO, USA ; 3 mg kg^{-1} i.v.) to block a possible release of vasodilator prostaglandins.

RESULTS

Intravenous injection of ET-1 produced a dose-dependent rise in MAP. At the highest dose MAP was increased by about 17 % with a concomitant decrease in HR by 9 %. ET-1 caused a pronounced, dose-dependent and long-lasting increase in bronchial blood flow. This was associated with a concomitant fall in bronchial vascular resistance by 15.6 ± 4 ($p < 0.05$) and 34.1 ± 4.8 % ($p < 0.01$) from baseline at doses of 45 pmol kg^{-1} and 450 pmol kg^{-1}, respectively, suggesting vasodilatation (Fig. 1). ET-1 also caused a slight decrease in nasal vascular resistance by 6.6 ± 1.6 and 10.0 ± 2.0 % at the same doses (Fig. 1). The vasodilator effect of ET-1 was not significantly attenuated after pretreatment with 3 mg.kg-1 of the cyclooxygenase inhibitor diclofenac. Pretreatment with systemic injection of capsaicin (50 mg kg^{-1}) two days before, did not modify the vascular response to ET-1 injections.

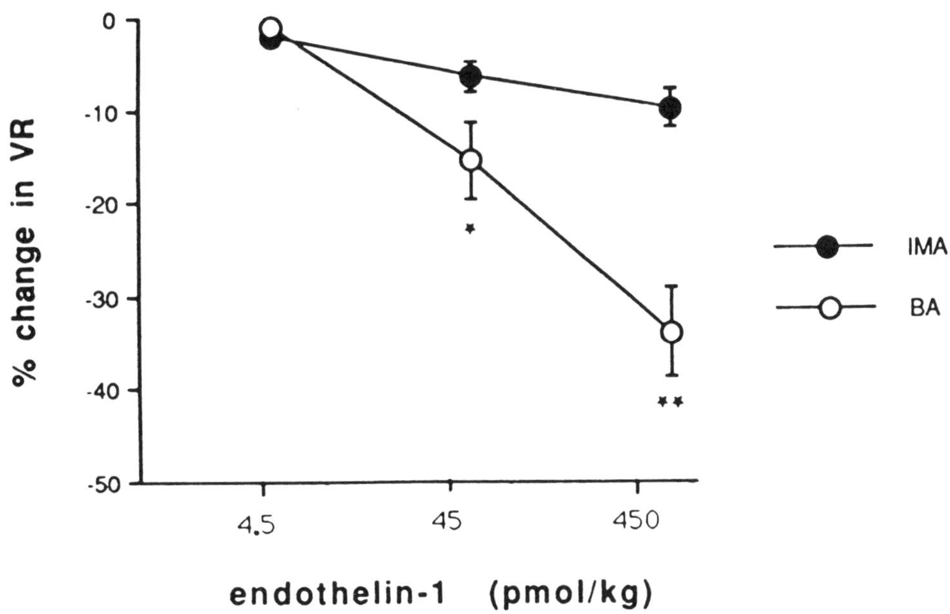

Figure 1. : Changes in bronchial (BA) and nasal (IMA) vascular resistance induced by increasing doses of endothelin-1 (4.5, 45 and 450 pmol kg^{-1}). Data are given as mean ± s.e. mean and expressed in per cent of control conditions. Significant differences from the basal values are calculated with Mann Whitney test ; * $p < 0.05$ and ** $p < 0.01$.

DISCUSSION

The present study demonstrates that in the pig, ET-1 produced a long-lasting, dose-related fall in vascular resistance in the vascular beds supplied by the bronchial artery i.e. ET-1 caused a clear-cut vasodilatation in this vascular
bed. ET-1 also caused an increase in systemic arterial blood pressure with a slight decrease in heart rate. Conversely, in the cat (Lippton et al., 1989) and the rat (Wright & Fozard, 1988) ET produced a fall in systemic blood pressure. These conflicting results may be explained by species differences in the cardiovascular effects of ET. The vascular effect of ET also depends on the organ studied. Intravenous administration of ET caused vasodilatation of certain vascular beds in cats (Lippton et al., 1989) whereas strong vasoconstriction has been observed in the pig renal artery (Pernow et al., 1989). We found ET-1 was a vasodilator agent of the bronchial circulation. Our findings confirm that ET-1 may be involved in the local regulation of peripheral vascular beds. The mechanism(s) whereby ET-1 causes vasodilatation in the bronchial mucosa is unclear.
Endothelial cells release various substances which are involved in vascular smooth muscle tone. Release of prostacyclin and thromboxane A2 from rat isolated lungs has been observed (De Nucci et al., 1988). In our study, however, the cyclooxygenase inhibitor, diclofenac, did not modify ET-1-induced vasodilatation of the bronchial circulation. It is, therefore, unlikely that ET-1 acts on the bronchial circulation through release of vasodilator prostanoïds. Although ET is the most potent vasoconstrictor peptide, it has also been shown that ET released endothelium-derived relaxing factor (EDRF) in the perfused mesentery of the rat (De Nucci et al., 1988). In the present study, the long-lasting vasodilatation observed in the bronchial circulation may be related to release of EDRF. However, further experiments should be performed with inhibitors of EDRF to confirm this hypothesis.
In addition, since capsaicin pretreatment had no effect on the vasodilator response, it is unlikely that neurogenic mechanisms involving tachykinin-containing C-fibers was at work in ET-1-evoked vasodilatation in the bronchial circulation.

CONCLUSION : ET-1 has potent vasodilator effects in the pig lower airway mucosa. Various mechanisms may explain the response e.g. release of EDRF. The selective effect of ET-1 on the bronchial circulation suggests that ET-1 is important in the regulation of regional vasomotor tone in the airway mucosa.

Acknowledgements : The present study was supported by grants from the Swedish Medical Research council (14 x 6554), the American Council for Tabacco Research, the Swedish Tabbaco Company, funds from the Karolinska Institute. We thank Miss Margareta Stensdother for expert technical assistance.

REFERENCES

De Nucci, G., Thomad, R., D'orleans-Juste, P., Antunes, E., Walder, C., Warner, T.D., & Vane, J.R. (1988). Pressor effects of circulating endothelin are limited by its removal in the pulmonary circulation and by the release of prostacyclin and endothelium-derived relaxing factor. Proc. Natl. Acad. Sci. 85, 9797-9800.

Furchgott, R.F. (1984). The role of endothelium in the responses of vascular smooth muscle to drugs. Ann. Rev. Pharmacol. Toxicol. 24, 175-197.

Lippton, H.L., Hauth, T.A., summer, W.R., & Hyman, A.L. (1989). Endothelin produces pulmonary vasoconstriction and systemic vasodilatation. J. Appl. Physiol. 66, 1008-1012.

Matran; R., Alving, K., & Lundberg, J.M. (1990). Cigarette smoke, nicotine and capsaicin induced vasodilatation in the pig respiratory mucoas. Br. J. Pharmacol., in press.

Pernow, J., Franco-Cerecceda, A., Matran, R., & Lundberg, J.M. (1989). Effect of Endothelin-1 on regional vascular resistances in the pig. J. Cardiovasc. Pharmacol., 13, S205-S206.

Vanhoutte, P.M. (1986). Epithelium-derived relaxing factor and bronchial reactivity. Am. Rev. Respir. Dis. 138, S24-S30.

Wright, C.E. & Fozard, J.R. (1988). Regional vasodilatation is a prominant feature of the haemodynamic response to endothelin in anaesthetized, spontaneously hypertensive rats. Eur. J. Pharmacol. 155, 201-203.

Yanagisawa, M., Kurihara, H., Kimura, S., Tomobe, M., Kobayashi, M., Mitsui, V., Yasaki, Y., Goto, K., and Masaki, T. (1988). *A novel potent vasoconstricteur peptide produced by vascular endothelial cells. Nature, 332, 411-415.

AAS 31:
Mediators in
Airway Hyperreactivity

PAF RECEPTORS IN GUINEA-PIG AND HUMAN LUNG

R.G. Goldie, K.E. Pedersen, P.J. Rigby and J.W. Paterson

Department of Pharmacology, University of Western Australia, Perth, Nedlands, 6009, Australia

SUMMARY: The autoradiographic distribution and density of specific binding sites for the PAF receptor antagonist [^{3}H]-WEB 2086 was assessed in non-diseased and asthmatic human lung and in guinea-pig airway tissue. In general, only very low levels of specific binding were detected in these tissues with no evidence for PAF receptors in airway smooth muscle. Asthma does not appear to involve significantly increased airway PAF receptor expression.

INTRODUCTION

Platelet activating factor (PAF) is an ether phospholipid mediator of inflammation which is capable of producing a number of biological effects which implicate it in the pathogenesis of asthma (Page, 1988). These effects include bronchoconstriction and the induction of bronchial hyperreactivity to inhaled spasmogens (Cuss et al., 1986). Specific binding sites for PAF have been detected in the guinea-pig and human lung membranes (Dent et al., 1989). The present study describes the autoradiographic distribution of specific binding sites for [^{3}H]-WEB 2086 in guinea-pig airway tissue as well as in human lung from non-diseased and from asthmatic subjects.

MATERIALS AND METHODS

Binding studies: Slide-mounted frozen sections (10 µm) of guinea-pig (SR/C Tricolour 400-500 g) peripheral lung were incubated at 22°C with [^{3}H]-WEB 2086 (1-160 nM) in Tris-HCl buffer (170 mM; pH 7.6) containing bovine serum albumin (0.25%) for 5-120 minutes. Non-specific binding was determined in the presence of non-radiolabelled WEB 2086 (10 µM) or PAF (10 µM). Sections were rapidly rinsed in buffer, wiped from slides with GF/A glass fibre filter paper and the radioactivity estimated by liquid scintillation counting.

Quantitative autoradiography: Human bronchial and peripheral lung tissue was obtained 2-10 h post mortem from 4 non-asthmatic (male, 11-74 years) and 4 asthmatic (3 male, 1 female, 19-63 years) subjects who had died during acute asthma attacks. Tracheal and peripheral lung tissue from guinea-pigs (SR/C Tricolour, 400-500 g) was also used. Slide-mounted frozen sections (10 µm) of tissue were incubated with [^{3}H]-WEB 2086 (80 nM) for 60 min at 22°C in Tris-HCl buffer. Non-specific binding was determined in the presence of 10 µM PAF. Tissue sections were rapidly washed, air-dried and opposed to nuclear track emulsion-coated (NTB-2) coverslips and placed in X-ray cassettes for 10 weeks for the production of autoradiograms. Specific grain densities over selected tissue types were determined using a computer-assisted image analysis system as described by Henry et al. (1990).

RESULTS

Binding studies: Specific binding of WEB 2086 in guinea-pig peripheral lung was both time (Fig 1a) and concentration (Fig 1b) dependent. Specific binding was maximal at approximately 60 min (Fig 1a). The dissociation constant (Kd) was approximately 25 µM as determined by interpolation (Fig 1b).

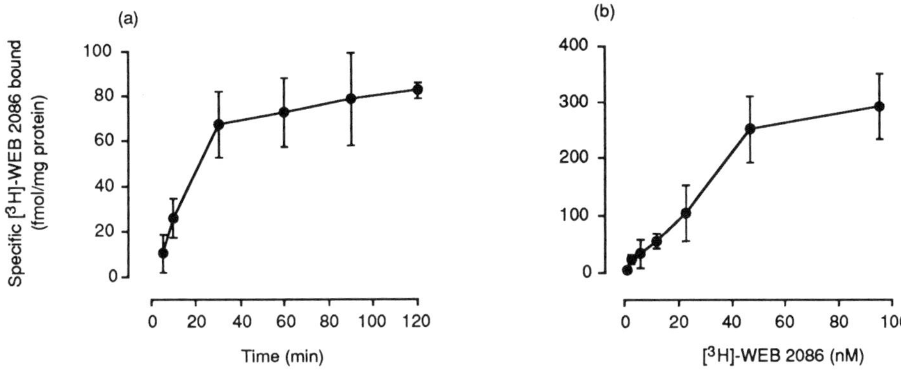

Figure 1. (a) Time-dependence ([^{3}H]-WEB 2086, 20 nM) (b) concentration-dependence of specific [^{3}H]-WEB 2086 binding.

Quantitative autoradiography: Very low numbers of specific autoradiographic grains were detected in the guinea-pig tracheal wall with the highest levels found in submucosal areas (Table I). Specific binding over airway smooth muscle was negligible.

Table I: [^{3}H]-WEB 2086 (80 nM) binding in guinea pig trachea

	Specific grain density (grains/10^4 μm^2)		
Animal No.	Smooth Muscle	Epithelium	Submucosa
1	*35.7	63.1	69.8
2	1.6	35.2	97.6
3	28.6	117.8	133.9
4	4.3	62.3	248.5
5	4.5	86.5	136.1
6	29.6	31.2	131.5
mean ± sem	17.4 ± 6.9	66.0 ± 14.5	136.2 ± 27.2

* Each value represents the mean estimate from 6 fields.

Very low specific grain densities were also detected in guinea-pig peripheral lung associated with alveolar wall tissue, the submucosa of bronchial walls and with some blood vessels.

The levels of specific binding in both non-diseased and asthmatic human peripheral lung were extremely low. Similarly, specific grain densities in human non-diseased and asthmatic bronchial smooth muscle and epithelium were negligible, although lower levels of binding were detected in submucosal gland tissue in non-asthmatic bronchi than in some asthmatic bronchi.

DISCUSSION

The number of PAF receptors is clearly very low in both guinea-pig and human lung tissue. The highest levels of specific [^{3}H]-WEB 2086 binding were associated with submucosal structures in guinea-pig trachea, perhaps involving sub-epithelial blood vessels of the bronchial circulation. In general, specific binding levels were lower in human than in guinea-pig lung structures. While some evidence was found for greater numbers of PAF receptors in asthmatic than in non-asthmatic bronchial submucosal gland tissue, asthma does not appear to involve significantly increased numbers of airway PAF receptors.

Acknowledgements: This work was supported by the National Health and Medical Research Council of Australia.

REFERENCES

Cuss, F.M., Dixon, C.M.S. and Barnes, P.J. (1986) Effects of inhaled platelet-activating factor on pulmonary function and bronchial responsiveness in man. Lancet, 2, 189-192.

Dent, F., Ukena, D., Sybrecht, G.W. and Barnes, P.J. (1989) [^{3}H]-WEB 2086 labels platelet activating factor receptors in guinea-pig and human lung. Eur. J. Pharmacol., 169, 313-316.

Henry, P.J., Rigby, P.J. and Goldie, R.G. (1990) Distribution of β_1 and β_2-adrenoceptors in mouse trachea and lung: a quantitative autoradiographic study. Br. J. Pharmacol., 99, 136-144.

Page, C.P. (1988) The role of platelet-activating factor in asthma. J. Allergy Clin. Immunol., 81, 144-152.

AAS 31:
Mediators in
Airway Hyperreactivity

SELECTIVE IMPLICATION OF THROMBOXANE A_2 AND PAF-ACETHER IN TWO GUINEA PIG ANAPHYLACTIC MODELS

C. Bertrand, E. Tschirhart and Y. Landry

Laboratoire de Neuroimmunopharmacologie, Université Louis Pasteur Strasbourg I, BP 24, 67401 ILLKIRCH Cedex, FRANCE.

SUMMARY: In an IgE and an IgG model of anaphylaxis in the guinea pig, we investigated the role of prostanoids and PAF-acether in the tracheal response *in vitro* to immunochallenge. Indomethacin (10^{-6}M) potentiated the antigen-induced contraction in both models suggesting the synthesis of relaxant prostaglandins during the anaphylactic phenomenon. UK-38,485 (10^{-5}M), a thromboxane (TxA_2) synthetase inhibitor, did not modify the tracheal response in the IgE model. In the IgG model, this drug reduced the response of the tracheal strips to antigen. Ro 19-3704 (10^{-6}M) and BN 52021 (10^{-5}M), two potent PAF antagonists, reduced antigen-induced contraction of the tracheal strips in the IgE model. These two drugs did not modify the contractile response in the IgG model. These results indicate that PAF-acether and TxA_2 play a role in the IgE and IgG model of anaphylaxis, respectively.

This study was designed to characterize the contributions of prostanoids and PAF-acether to antigen-induced contraction in tracheal preparations from actively sensitized guinea pigs. Most studies agree that contractile responses are the results of the actions of histamine and leukotrienes (Adams and Lichtenstein, 1979). Release of thromboxane A_2 (TxA_2) and PAF-acether has also been demonstrated during anaphylaxis (Chung et al., 1986; Fitzgerald et al., 1986). In order to ascertain the influence of antibody type mediating the response, studies were carried out in IgE and IgG models of anaphylaxis.

MATERIALS AND METHODS

Guinea-pig sensitizations, tissue preparations and experimental protocols have been described previously (Bertrand et al., 1989). UK-38,485 was obtained from Pfizer (Sandwich, England), BN 52021 from IHB-IPSEN (Le Plessis-Robinson, France), Ro 19-3704 from Hoffmann-LaRoche (Basel, Switzerland) and indomethacin from Merck, Sharp & Dohme (Riom, France). The parameters measured in this study were: the peak of contraction (5 min after the addition of antigen) ; the protracted phase of contraction (30 min after the addition of antigen). Results (in mg of contraction) are expressed as means ± S.E.M of 9 experiments. Unpaired Student's t-test was used to determine the significance of differences between mean values in control and test tissues, with a 95% confidence level (indicated by *).

RESULTS

Addition of antigen induced a contractile response in both sensitization models. Indomethacin (10^{-6}M), potentiated the antigen-induced contractile response, increasing the peak of contraction (5 min) and enhancing the protracted phase of the response (30 min) in both sensitization models (Fig. 1). The TxA2 synthetase inhibitor, UK-38,485 (10^{-5}M), had no effect on tracheal contraction in the IgE model.(Fig. 1A). In the IgG model, this compound inhibited both phases of contraction (Fig. 1B). In the IgE model, the PAF antagonist, Ro 19-3704 (10^{-6}M), decreased the onset (5 min) and the protracted phases (30 min) of the contraction of the tracheal strips (Fig. 2A). In the IgG model, Ro 19-3704 had no effect (Fig. 2B). BN 52021 (10^{-5}M) displayed the same activity profile as Ro 19-3704, although it was less potent in the IgE model (Fig. 2A and 2B).

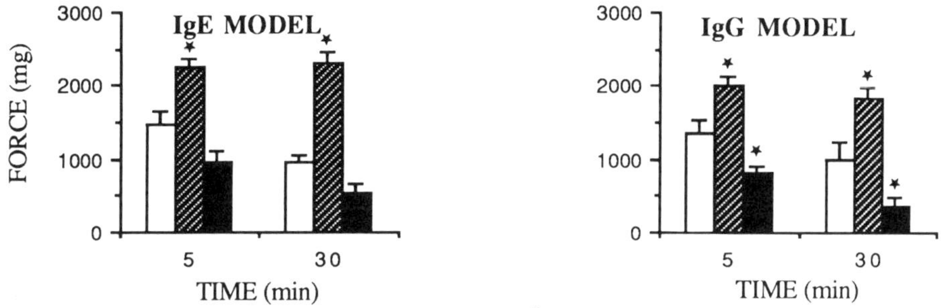

Figure 1 : Effect of indomethacin (10^{-6}M, hatched column) and UK-38,485 (10^{-5}M, solid column) on the response to ovalbumin (10^{-5}g/ml) compared to untreated tracheal strips (open column).

DISCUSSION

In this study, we provide evidence for a direct participation in anaphylactic response of PAF-acether and prostanoids, whose release and/or synthesis are strongly dependent upon the sensitization procedure. Histamine and leukotrienes are the main mediators of antigen-induced bronchospasm in guinea pig sensitized to produce IgE and IgG antibodies (Andersson, 1982; Bertrand et al., 1989). The role of cyclooxygenase products in the anaphylactic reaction, however, remains controversial. Indomethacin potentiated the antigen-induced IgE- and IgG-mediated tracheal contractions.

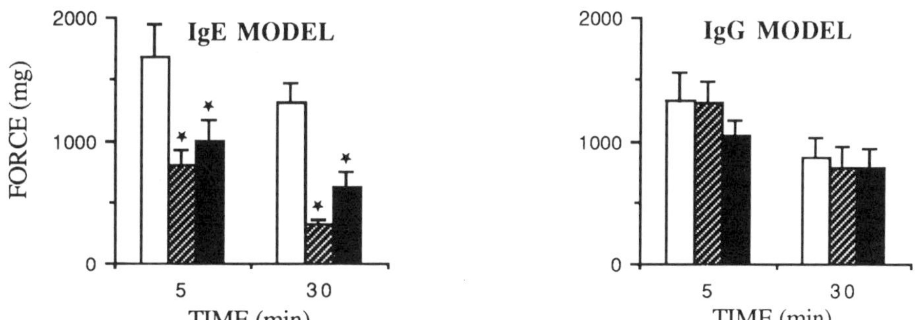

Figure 2 : Effect of Ro 19-3704 (10^{-6}M, hatched columns) and BN 52021 (10^{-5}M, solid columns) on the response to ovalbumin (10^{-5} g/ml) compared to untreated tracheal strips (open columns).

These results and other reports indicate that this effect is due to the inhibition of relaxing prostaglandin synthesis (Andersson, 1982). The potentiating effect of indomethacin might be also related to a redirection of arachidonic acid metabolism through the lipoxygenase pathway (Undem et al., 1987). In the IgG model, the inhibitory effect of UK-38,485 suggests that TxA_2 is involved in the onset and maintenance of the tracheal contraction. This result suggests a differential release of TxA_2 in the two models of anaphylaxis. The effects of two PAF receptor antagonists, BN 52021 and Ro 19-3704, suggest that PAF is involved in the antigen-induced contractile response in the IgE model only. These results indicate that PAF may be released during airway anaphylaxis as previously suggested by Darius et al. (1986). In conclusion, our study shows that, in addition to the known role of histamine and leukotrienes, thromboxane A_2 and PAF are implicated in the IgG and IgE models of anaphylaxis respectively.

REFERENCES

Adams, G.K.III & Lichtenstein, L. (1979) In vitro studies of antigen-induced bronchospasm : effect of antihistamine and SRS-A antagonists on response of sensitized guinea-pig and human airways to antigen. J. Immunol. 122, 555-562.

Andersson, P. (1982) Effects of inhibitors of anaphylactic mediators in two models of bronchial anaphylaxis in anaesthetized guinea-pigs. Br. J. Pharmacol. 77, 301-307.

Bertrand, C., Tschirhart, E. & Landry, Y. (1989) Nedocromil sodium inhibits IgE- and IgG-related antigen-induced contraction in guinea-pig trachea. Int. Arch. Allergy Appl. Immunol. 88, 439-446.

Chung, K.F., Aizawa, A. Becker, A.B., Frick, O., Gold, W.M. and Nadel, J.A. (1986) Inhibition of antigen-induced airway hyperresponsiveness by a thromboxane synthetase inhibitor (OKY-046) in allergic dogs. Am. Rev. Resp. Dis. 134, 258-261.

Darius, H., Smith, J.B. & Lefer, A.M. (1986) Inhibition of the platelet activating factor mediated component of guinea pig anaphylaxis by receptor antagonists. Int. Arch. Allergy Appl. Immunol. 80, 369-375.

Fitzgerald, M.F., Moncada, S. & Parente, L. (1986) The anaphylactic release of platelet activating factor from perfused guinea pig lungs. Br. J. Pharmacol. 88, 149-153.

Undem, B.J., Pickett, W.C. & Adams, G.K.III (1987) Antigen-induced sulfidopeptide leukotriene release from the guinea pig superfused trachea. Eur. J. Pharmacol. 142, 31-37.

AAS 31:
Mediators in
Airway Hyperreactivity

EFFECTS OF A NOVEL PAF ANTAGONIST, E6123, ON PAF-INDUCED BIOLOGICAL RESPONSES

H. Tsunoda, Y. Sakuma, K. Harada, K. Muramoto, S. Katayama, T. Horie, N. Shimomura, R. Clark, S. Miyazawa, K. Okano, Y. Machida, K. Katayama, I. Yamastu

Tsukuba Research Lab., Eisai Co., Ltd., 1-3, Tokodai 5-chome, Tsukuba-shi, Ibaraki 300-26, Japan

SUMMARY: E6123 is a new member of the benzodiazepine class of PAF antagonists. Although it has similar activity *in vitro* to the two representative antagonists WEB2347 and Y24180, *in vivo* it is far more active than these compounds. Thus E6123 was effective in inhibiting dose-dependently PAF-induced bronchoconstriction when administered orally or intravenously (IC_{50} 1.0 and 1.3 μg/Kg, respectively, at 3 hr), and had a minimum effective dose of 10 μg/Kg and 3 μg/Kg, respectively, against PAF-induced hematoconcentration and edema at 3 hr after oral administration. Furthermore, E6123 protects mice from PAF-induced death dose-dependently (ED_{50} 7 μg/Kg at 3 hr). In conclusion, E6123 should prove valuable in pharmacological and clinical research into the roles of PAF, and in therapy of diseases such as asthma, in which PAF is assumed to play a pathological role.

INTRODUCTION

Platelet-activating factor (PAF) is known to be associated with bronchoconstriction, chemotaxis, airway secretion, microvascular leakage and bronchial hyperreactivity. These effects may be relevant to asthma and it has therefore been suggested that selective antagonists of PAF may be beneficial for the treatment of asthma and bronchial hyperreactivity. (S)-(+)-6-(2-Chlorophenyl)-3-cyclopropanecarbonyl-8,11-dimethyl-2,3,4,5-tetrahydro-8H-pyrido[4',3':4,5]thieno-[3,2-f][1,2,4]triazolo[4,3-a][1,4]diazepine, E6123, is a PAF antagonist newly synthesized in our laboratory. In the present study we have examined its effects on PAF-induced responses in a variety of in vitro, ex vivo and in vivo test systems.

MATERIALS AND METHODS

In vitro experiments Platelet aggregation: Platelet-rich plasma was incubated with the test compound for 3 min at 37°C before the addition of PAF (final concentration 50, 1 and 30 ng/ml for human, guinea pig and dog, respectively). The aggregation induced by PAF was followed by using a aggregometer (Niko Bioscience). ^{3}H-PAF binding to platelets: Platelets were preincubated with ^{3}H-PAF (0.6-1 nM, Amersham) for 6 min at 37°C. The reaction was terminated by adding cold washing solution. Platelets were isolated by vacuum filtration on glass filters. The reactivity on the glass was measured.
Ex vivo experiments E6123 was administered orally to guinea pig (Hartley) or dog (beagle) and platelets were taken at various times after administration. Platelet aggregation was assayed by the method described above. ^{3}H-PAF binding to platelets in guinea pig was assayed according to the method of Kloprogge and Akkerman (1984).
In vivo experiments PAF-induced bronchoconstriction: Guinea pigs were anesthetized by intraperitoneal injection of urethane (1.25 g/Kg) and prepared for recording of bronchospasm according to the method of Konzett and Rossler (1940), then challenged with either sequential administrations of PAF (100 ng/Kg, i.v.) with a 30 min interval or by inhalation of aerosolized PAF (1 mg/ml, 30 sec). The inhibitory effects of the test compounds on the bronchoconstriction induced by the second PAF injection or PAF inhalation were evaluated. Hematoconcentration: The blood was collected by cardiac puncture at 10 min after PAF injection (300 ng/Kg) in conscious guinea pigs. The hematocrit was determined by using a hematocrit reader after centrifugation. Edema: The tracheal edema was evaluated at 5 min after PAF injection (100 ng/Kg) according to the method of Evans et al. (1988). Mortality: Mortality of mice (ICR) was determined 24 hr after

PAF injection (80 $\mu g/Kg$) according to the method of Young et al.(1985). Test compounds were administered orally at 3 hr before the PAF injection, unless otherwise stated.

RESULTS AND DISCUSSION

Table I shows the PAF antagonistic activity of E6123 and other PAF antagonists on ^3H-PAF binding to the platelets and on PAF-induced platelet aggregation. In these in vitro models, E6123 was more potent than WEB2086 and WEB2170 and as potent as WEB2347 and Y24180.

E6123 at 3 $\mu g/Kg$ caused complete inhibition of ex vivo PAF-induced platelet aggregation in guinea pigs at 1.5 hr after administration of E6123. This 100% inhibition lasted for at least 8 hr and a significant inhibition was still observed even at 24 hr. The receptor occupancy was about 80%, 56% and 38% at 3, 24 and 48 hr, respectively, after administration (data not shown). In dogs, E6123 (3 $\mu g/Kg$ and 10 $\mu g/Kg$) also inhibited ex vivo PAF-induced platelet aggregation dose-dependently (data not shown).

Between 1.5 and 8 hr after administration of E6123, more than 90% inhibition of PAF-induced bronchoconstriction was observed, and the effect gradually reduced over 36 hr (data not shown).

Bronchoconstriction induced by injection of PAF was inhibited dose-dependently by oral or intravenous administration of E6123 at similar doses (data not shown).

Table I Inhibitory effects of test compounds on ^3H-PAF binding to washed platelets and platelet aggregation

Test method	Animal	Unit	E6123	WEB2086	WEB2170 (nM)	WEB2347	Y24180
^3H-PAF binding to platelet	human	IC_{50}	2.6	46.3	14.1	1.4	1.1
	g.p.	IC_{50}	3.0	7.7	11.9	1.5	n.d.
Platelet aggregation	human	IC_{50}	10.1	35.4	20.1	18.6	24.3
	g.p.	IC_{50}	14.7	60.6	44.5	19.6	15.1
	beagle	IC_{50}	16.0	58.8	34.9	23.1	52.0

g.p.: guinea pig n.d.: not determined

Table II Anti-PAF effects of E6123 and other PAF antagonists

Test method	Animal	Time (hr)	Unit	Test compounds (μg/Kg) (1)	(2)	(3)	(4)	(5)
Bronchoconstriction (PAF i.v.)	g.p.	1.5	ED_{50}	2.4	65	12.2	>10	15
		3		1.0	400	n.d.	11	17
		8		0.8	n.d.	26.0	11	20
Bronchoconstriction (PAF inhalation)	g.p.	1.5	ED_{50}	4.0	700	19.0	n.d.	n.d.
		3		1.3	n.d.	n.d.	26	12
Hematoconcentration (PAF i.v.)	g.p.	3	MED	10	n.d.	n.d.	100	100
Edema (PAF i.v.)	g.p.	3	MED	3	n.d.	n.d.	100	100
Mortality (PAF i.v.)	mouse	3	ED_{50}	7	3000	n.d.	250	40

(1) E6123 (2) WEB2086 (3) WEB2170 (4) WEB2347 (5) Y24180
Time: time after oral administration,
n.d.: not determined, g.p.: guinea pig

Table II shows the effects of E6123 and other antagonists on PAF-induced bronchoconstriction, hematoconcentration, edema and mortality. E6123 was the most potent of the PAF antagonists examined in *in vivo* models of PAF-induced effects. E6123 was more potent than the representative potent antagonists, WEB2347 and Y24180, although the PAF-antagonistic activities of the three compounds *in vitro* were similar. This suggests that the pharmacokinetics of E6123 are much better than those of WEB2347 and Y24180. In conclusion, the present results suggest that E6123 may be beneficial for the treatment of asthma, in which PAF is assumed to be involved.

REFERENCES

Evans, T.W., Dent, G., Rogers, D.F., Aursudkij, B., Chung, K.F., and Barnes, P.J. (1988), Br. J. Pharmacol. 94, 164-168

Kloprogge, E. and Akkerman, J.W.N. (1984), Biochem.J. 223, 901-909

Konzett, H. and Rossler, R. (1940), Arch. Exp. Path. Pharmacok. 195, 71-74

Young, J.M., Malcony, P.J., Jubb, S.N., and Clark, J.S. (1985), Prostaglandins 30, 545-551

AAS 31:
Mediators in
Airway Hyperreactivity

EFFECTS OF A NOVEL PAF ANTAGONIST, E6123, ON PASSIVE ANAPHYLAXIS

Y. Sakuma, H. Tsunoda, S. Katayama, K. Harada, H. Obaishi, M. Shirato, K. Yamada, S. Miyazawa, K. Okano, Y. Machida, K. Katayama, I. Yamastu

Tsukuba Research Lab., Eisai Co., Ltd., 1-3, Tokodai 5-chome, Tsukuba-shi, Ibaraki 300-26, Japan

SUMMARY: E6123 inhibited antigen-induced bronchoconstriction, the development of bronchial hyperreactivity and eosinophil infiltration in the airway in passively sensitized guinea pigs and protected mice from anaphylactic death. The inhibitory effects of E6123 on anaphylactic response were very potent compared with those of WEB 2347 and Y-24180.

INTRODUCTION

The pathophysiology of asthma is characterized by bronchial smooth muscle constriction in the early phase and excessive mucus production, bronchial edema and inflammation followed by accumulation of inflammatory cells in the airways in the late phase. It has been suggested that platelet-activating factor (PAF) may be an important mediator of asthma and inflammation (Vargaftig and Braquet, 1987; Page, 1987). Since PAF is assumed to mimic most of the pathophysiological features of asthma, PAF antagonists seem to be promising drugs for therapy of asthma. The search for specific PAF antagonists has led us to the synthesis of E6123, (S)-(+)-6-(2-chlorophenyl)-3-cyclopropanecarbonyl-8,11-dimethyl-2,3,4,5-tetrahydro-8H-pyrido[4',3':4,5]thieno-[3,2-f][1,2,4]triazolo[4,3-a][1,4]diazepine.

MATERIALS AND METHODS

Respiratory function: Male Hartley guinea pigs (Japan SLC, Inc.; 300-500 g body weight) were intravenously injected with 5 ml/Kg homologous anti-ovalbumin serum (1/10 diluted, 48 hr PCA titer 1/12,000) 17-24 hr prior to the antigen challenge. An antigen (ovalbumin, Ag; 1 mg/Kg) was injected to induce broncho-constriction in passively sensitized guinea pigs that had been pretreated with antihistamine (pyrilamine; 2.5 mg/Kg, i.v.), BW755c (2 mg/Kg, i.v.) and propranolol (0.05 mg/Kg, i.v.). As an index of pulmonary function, respiratory flow was measured with a pneumotachograph, a differential pressure transducer and a recorder (Nihon Kohden, Japan) in spontaneously breathing guinea pigs. Bronchoconstriction was also induced by Ag inhalation (2 mg/ml during 1 min) in passively sensitized guinea pigs that had been pretreated with pyrilamine and propranolol. Airway obstruction was measured according to the method of Konzett and Rossler (1940). In bronchial hyperreactivity, guinea pigs that had been pretreated with pyrilamine were exposed to an aerosol of Ag (10 mg/ml for 10 min) and 24 hr after Ag exposure respiratory flow was measured by the method described above. Bronchial reactivity was assessed by i.v. administration of histamine (1-50 μg/Kg).

Eosinophil infiltration: Guinea pigs that had been pretreated with pyrilamine were exposed to an aerosol of Ag (0.3 mg/ml for 10 min) and 24 hr after Ag exposure, they were killed by an overdose of pentobarbital. Phosphate-buffered saline (8 ml) was flushed into the lungs via a tracheal cannula. The fluid was withdrawn immediately. This procedure was repeated a total of 6 times and the lavage fluid was collected. Total cell counts were performed with a SYSMEX E3000 (Toa Medical Electronics, Japan) and eosinophil counts were performed in an eosinophil counter after staining with Hinkelman's solution.

Anaphylactic shock in mice: Male ICR strain mice (Charles River Japan Inc.; 40-52 g body weight) were intravenously injected with 10 ml/Kg rabbit anti-ovalbumin serum (1/10 diluted, 6 hr guinea pig PCA titer 1/24,000) 2 hr prior to the i.v. Ag challenge (5 mg/Kg with 0.05 mg/Kg propranolol). The survival rate was recorded. In this experiment the lethality was more than 95%.

RESULTS AND DISCUSSION

Table I shows the minimum effective dose of E6123 and other PAF antagonists on antigen-induced bronchoconstriction, bronchial hyperreactivity, eosinophil infiltration in guinea pigs and ED_{50} of the PAF antagonists on mortality in mice. E6123 was far more potent than the representative PAF antagonists WEB 2086, WEB 2347 (Boehringer Ingelheim) and Y-24180 (Yoshitomi Pharmaceutical Co.) in several passive anaphylaxis models. E6123 inhibited Ag inhalation-induced bronchoconstriction and eosinophil infiltration by only 50% at the maximum dose used, although the complete inhibition by E6123 was seen in the case of i.v. administration of Ag. This result seems to be based on another mechanism and sequence of events.

Table I Effects of E6123 and other PAF antagonists[a] on passive anaphylaxis

Test method	Animal	E6123	WEB2086	WEB2347	Y-24180
Bronchoconstriction (MED[b]) (Ag i.v.)	g.p.[c]	3	(300)	30	30
Bronchoconstriction (MED) (Ag inhalation)	g.p.	3	n.d.[d]	1,000	>1,000
Bronchial hyperreactivity (MED) (Ag inhalation)	g.p.	30	(>100,000)	10,000	>10,000
Eosinophil infiltration (MED) (Ag inhalation)	g.p.	300	n.d.	>10,000	>10,000
Mortality (ED_{50}) (Ag i.v.)	mouse	7	(4,800)	270	205

[a] The drugs (μg/Kg) were administered orally 3 hr prior to the Ag challenge except for WEB2086 (1 or 1.5 hr).
[b] Minimum effective dose
[c] Guinea pig
[d] Not determined

The specificity of E6123 as a PAF antagonist was clarified by the following in vitro results. The IC_{50} value of E6123 on PAF-induced platelet aggregation was 10.1 nM. At 10 μM, E6123 showed no effect on ADP-induced platelet aggregation, acetylcholine and/or histamine-induced contraction, benzodiazepine receptor binding, and cyclooxygenase, lipoxygenase, thromboxane synthetase and phospholipase A_2 activities. Collagen-induced platelet aggregation was inhibited with an IC_{50} of 19 μM E6123.

E6123, which is a specific and potent PAF antagonist, inhibited several anaphylactic reactions in this experiment. Furthermore it was suggested that arachidonic acid metabolites are generated after i.v. administration of PAF in guinea pigs (Lewis et al., 1984), and the contraction of tracheal smooth muscle in rat was potentiated by pretreatment with PAF (Chand et al., 1986). It has been suggested that PAF may be an important mediator of asthma and inflammation.

CONCLUSION: The pharmacological effect of E6123 in anaphylaxis induced by Ag exposure is greater than that of the representative potent antagonists WEB 2347 and Y-24180, though the IC_{50} of E6123 in the PAF receptor binding assay was similar to those of WEB 2347 and Y-24180. These results suggest that E6123 may be useful in the therapy of airway hyperreactivity, in which PAF is assumed to be involved.

REFERENCES

Chand, N., Mahoney, T.P., Diamantis, W., and Sofia, R.D. (1986), Eur. J. Pharmacol. 123, 315-317

Konzett, H., and Ressler, R. (1940), Arch. Exp. Path. Parmak. 195, 71-74

Lewis, A.J., Dervinis, A., and Chang, J. (1984), Agents and Actions 15(5/6), 636-642

Page, C.P. (1987), Int. J. Tissue React. 9, 27-32

Vargaftig, B.B., and Braquet, P. (1987), Br. Med. Bull. 43, 312-335

AAS 31:
Mediators in
Airway Hyperreactivity

PUTATIVE ROLE OF EPITHELIAL DERIVED FACTORS IN AIRWAY SMOOTH MUSCLE REACTIVITY

D. Raeburn

Rhone-Poulenc (UK) Ltd., Biological Research, Dagenham Research Centre, Dagenham, Essex, RM10 7XS, England

SUMMARY: Until recently the contractile actions of asthma mediators have been examined in vitro without consideration of the modulatory role of the associated epithelial cells. Removal of the epithelium in vitro augments contraction and reduces relaxation to several bronchoactive agents and bioassay experiments have shown that the protective effects of the epithelium can be transferred to denuded preparations. It now seems likely that one or more epithelial-associated factors eg EpDRF and PGE_2 have a protective role in controlling airway contractility. These findings may be important in asthmatics in vivo since there may be some correlation between epithelial damage/loss and airway hyperreactivity. The identity of EpDRF remains unknown but it does not appear to be a prostanoid and is distinct pharmacologically from EDRF found in blood vessels.

INTRODUCTION

The airway smooth muscle constrictor effects of the putative mediators of asthma when studied in vitro have not, until recently, taken into account the influence of the epithelial cells present in these isolated preparations. The epithelium has generally been regarded as having a passive barrier role in the airways removing irritant substances by ciliary activity and preventing access of noxious stimuli to the underlying smooth muscle, nerve endings and proinflammatory cells. Since the demonstration that vascular endothelial cells release the smooth muscle relaxant endothelium-derived relaxant factor (EDRF, see review by Furchgott, 1984) and that in asthmatics there is epithelial cell damage which may be correlated with the degree of severity of airway hyperreactivity, a new interest has emerged in the possible role of the epithelium in regulating airway reactivity in asthma. This review will discuss the involvement of the epithelium in muscle reactivity in vivo and in vitro and consider the evidence for the role of epithelium derived relaxant or inhibitory "factors".

THE EPITHELIUM IN ASTHMA

In histological studies of asthmatic lung obtained post mortem, a prominent feature is the widespread damage to the respiratory epithelium (Dunnill, 1960; Filley et al., 1982). The greatest degree of damage was seen in patients dying during an acute episode of asthma whereas little or no damage to the epithelium was evident in tissues from a non-asthmatic control group. Large numbers of eosinophils and released major basic protein (MBP) were associated with the areas of epithelial damage (Filley et al., 1982). Other early reports demonstrated that during exacerbations of asthma large numbers of epithelial cells can be found in the sputum of asthmatics (Sanerkin & Evans, 1965). The epithelial cells presumably had become detached from the airways.

Recently some attempts have been made to determine the condition of the airway epithelium in living asthmatics by examining bronchial biopsy material. Some attempt has been made to correlate the degree of epithelial damage with the severity of bronchial hyperreactivity. The findings are summarized in Table I. At both light and electron microscopic levels varying degrees of epithelial damage including marked desquamation was commonly seen in biopsies of asthmatic lung.

Table I COMPARISON OF BRONCHIAL BIOPSY DATA FROM ASTHMATIC AND CONTROL SUBJECTS

EPITHELIAL DAMAGE CONTROL	ASTHMATIC	BHR ASTHMATIC	CORRELATION	REFERENCE
-	+/+++	HIST	NONE FOUND	LAITINEN et al.(1985)
-	-/+++	MCh	n. d.	ELIA et al. (1988)
-	+++	MCh	r = 0.68 p < 0.015	BEASLEY et al. (1988)
-	+++	MCh	r = 0.67 p < 0.001	JEFFERY et al. (1989)
-/++	+/++	MCh	NONE FOUND	LOZEWICZ et al. (1990)

-, no damage +, varying degrees of damage n.d., not determined
HIST, histamine MCh, methacholine BHR, bronchial hyperreactivity

Normal epithelium was seen only in the non-asthmatic control tissues (Laitinen et al.,1985; Elia et al., 1988; Beasley et al., 1988; Jeffery et al., 1989). On the other hand Lozewicz et al.(1990) found epithelial damage in control and asthmatic subjects. Significant correlation between the degree of epithelial damage and bronchial hyperreactivity was demonstrated by Beasley et al. (1988) and Jeffery et al. (1989) whereas no correlation was found by Laitinen et al. (1985) or Lozewicz et al. (1990). Clearly more comparative studies are required to resolve these differences.

EPITHELIUM REMOVAL IN VITRO

The effect of epithelium removal on the reactivity of the underlying airway smooth muscle in vitro was first reported by Flavahan et al. (1985). Since then several reviews dealing with various aspects of this phenomenon have been published (Vanhoutte, 1987, 1988; Fedan et al., 1988; Allegra et al.,

1989; Raeburn, 1990; Goldie et al., 1990). Following epithelium removal there is generally an augmented contractility to spasmogens and a reduced relaxant effect to smooth muscle relaxants (Fig. 1). Not all bronchoactive agents are affected, eg. epithelium removal has no effect on responses to KCl or salbutamol (see review by Fedan et al., 1988). Species differences and regional variation in the effects of epithelium removal also can be seen.

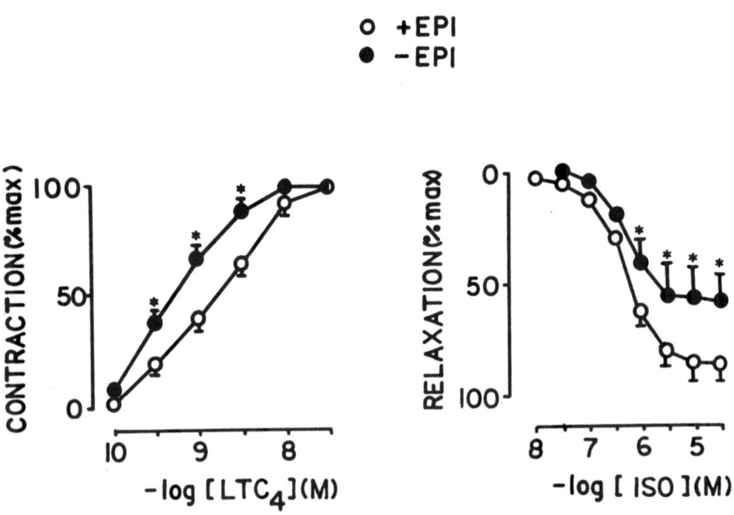

Fig. 1. Effect of epithelium removal on airway smooth muscle responses to LTC_4 (guinea pig) and isoprenaline (canine, redrawn from Flavahan et al., 1985)., $^*p < 0.05$

IS THERE AN EPITHELIUM-DERIVED RELAXANT FACTOR?

Several explanations including loss of a diffusion barrier, loss of a site of metabolism and the loss of eicosanoid and non-eicosanoid relaxant "factors" have been proposed to explain the modulatory effects of epithelium. As yet there is insufficient evidence to propose a unifying hypothesis and all mechanisms may play some major or minor role depending on the circumstances involved.

LOSS OF A DIFFUSION BARRIER

The increased airway reactivity to antigen in epithelium denuded tissues (Hay et al., 1986, 1987) may in part be due to the loss of the barrier actions of the epithelium (Undem et al., 1987) facilitating greater access to the submucosal mast cells. However, this explanation is not tenable in the case of augmented responses to nerve stimulation in denuded tissues where the transmitter is released directly onto the muscle and hence its action is not dependent on diffusion through the mucosa (Flavahan et al., 1985). It is also difficult to reconcile the loss of a diffusion barrier with the decreased reactivity to isoprenaline in canine airways (Flavahan et al., 1985) and the conversion of the relaxant response to arachidonic acid to contraction on epithelium removal (Nijkamp & Folkerts, 1987; Farmer et al., 1987a,b).

LOSS OF A SITE OF METABOLISM

While the increased contractility to acetylcholine in epithelium-denuded tissues is not explained by the loss of cholinesterase activity (Flavahan et al., 1985) loss of sites of epithelial metabolism may play a role in the altered reactivity to several other agents in intact compared with

Table II COMPOUNDS AFFECTED BY ALTERED UPTAKE OR METABOLISM FOLLOWING EPITHELIUM REMOVAL

SUBSTANCE	EFFECT OF ALTERED METABOLISM
ISOPRENALINE	INCREASED RELAXATION (loss of COMT, MAO activity)
ADENOSINE	INCREASED RELAXATION (loss of ADENOSINE DEAMINASE)
VIP	INCREASED RELAXATION (loss of NEP)
SUBSTANCE P, NEUROKININ A,B	INCREASED CONTRACTION (loss of NEP, CYCLOOXYGENASE)
ARACHIDONIC ACID	CONTRACTION (loss of CYCLOOXYGENASE)

COMT, catechol-o-methyl transferase MAO, monoamine oxidase
NEP, neutral endopeptidase (enkephalinase) VIP, vasoactive intestinal peptide

denuded tissues (Fedan et al., 1988; Allegra et al., 1989; Raeburn, 1990; Goldie et al., 1990). The data suggesting alterations in contractility resulting from epithelial metabolism are summarized in Table II. Possibly the most important example of epithelial metabolic activity is the conversion of arachidonic acid-induced relaxation to contraction in denuded tissues (Nijkamp & Folkerts, 1987; Farmer et al, 1987a,b; Raeburn, 1990). This suggests that under normal circumstances the epithelium metabolizes arachidonic acid to a relaxant (protective?) substance. This subject will be discussed later. Another important finding is that in human tissues epithelial associated NEP is important in reducing contractility to the neurokinins (Naline et al., 1989).

EPITHELIUM-DERIVED RELAXANT FACTOR (EpDRF)

The majority of studies reporting an altered airway reactivity following epithelium removal in vitro ascribe this finding to the loss of an endogenous relaxant or (more correctly) an inhibitory factor which acts to reduce airway smooth muscle contractility. The factor is now most commonly referred to as Epithelium-Derived Relaxant Factor (EpDRF) but the alternative Epithelium-Derived Inhibitory Factor (EpDIF) is also used. The findings from early studies provided no direct evidence to support the existence of epithelium-associated factors. It is only the development of bioassay procedures that has strengthened the argument in favour of the existence of specific relaxant factors produced by and released from the airway epithelium.

Using a cascade bioassay system where epithelium-denuded airway smooth muscle preparations from guinea pig or dog were superfused with physiological salt solution which had been passed through tube preparations of airways containing the epithelium, Flavahan & Vanhoutte (1985) and Vanhoutte (1987, 1988) have demonstrated an epithelium-dependent relaxation. This suggests the transfer of a factor from the intact to the denuded preparations. The authors have stated that the relaxations obtained were variable and suggest that release of the factor normally would be directed towards the smooth muscle away from the airway lumen thus reducing the concentration of EpDRF effectively available for transfer. This, and the predicted short biological half-life of EpDRF, could account for the failure of other studies to demonstrate factor release (Holroyde, 1986; Undem et al., 1987). A "sandwich" type assay where contractility is measured in a denuded tissue which is tied to an epithelium intact tissue also has been used sucessfully to demonstrate transfer of an epithelium-associated relaxant factor (Tschirhart et al., 1987). Here the epithelium-dependent relaxation to arachidonic acid was demonstrated in denuded strips which were attached to intact tissues. Unfortunately other attempts at demonstrating EpDRF release using this technique have been less successful (see Fedan et al., 1988).

The problems of the cascade superfusion and sandwich

bioassay have been largely overcome by the introduction of the co-axial bioassay technique. Here the assay tissue (the "acceptor") is surrounded by a tube of airway smooth muscle containing the epithelium (the "donor"). Diffusion of relaxant factor away from the assay tissue should therefore be more limited. Suitable acceptor tissues have included rat aorta, rat anococcygeus and guinea-pig trachealis. The non airway smooth muscle acceptors have the advantage that they can be contracted by phenylephrine (which has minimal effects on airway smooth muscle) and epithelium-dependent relaxation rather than reduced contractility can be measured.

Using co-axial bioassay, EpDRF release has been shown to occur following tissue stimulation with muscarinic agonists,

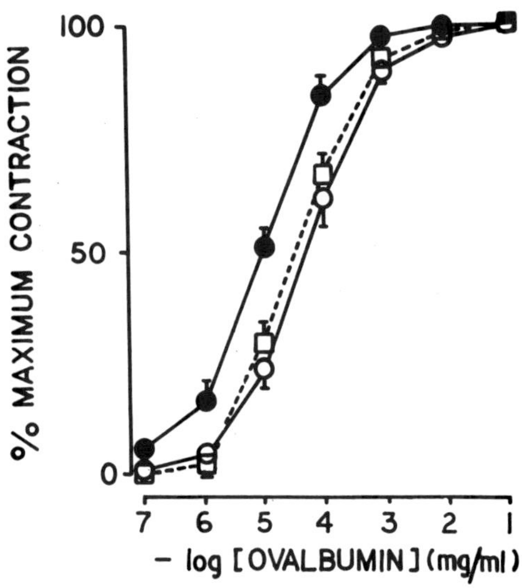

Fig. 2. Concentration-response curves to ovalbumin in co-axial bioassay, guinea-pig trachealis. Responses were recorded from the acceptor tissues. Both epithelium containing (○), both denuded (●), denuded acceptor inside intact donor tube (□). Redrawn from Hay et al. (1987).

histamine, arachidonic acid and, in sensitized animals, ovalbumin (Ilhan & Sahin, 1986; Hay et al., 1987; Farmer et al., 1987b; Guc et al., 1988; Fernandes et al., 1989; Hay et al., 1989). The modulatory role of the epithelium on responses to antigen challenge in co-axial bioassay is shown in Fig. 2. EpDRF release from human bronchial epithelium has now been demonstrated (Fernandes et al., 1989).

The evidence obtained from the bioassay studies suggests that EpDRF is unlikely to be a prostanoid since, where tested, indomethacin did not prevent its activity (Ilhan & Sahin, 1986; Guc et al., 1988; Fernandes et al., 1989). In contrast to these findings in the coaxial bioassay systems, indomethacin blocked the relaxant activity to arachidonic acid in the sandwich studies (Tschirhart et al., 1987). It is probable that this is due to a direct effect of the cyclooxygenase inhibitor on the generation of PGE_2 from the exogenously applied arachidonic acid and not on EpDRF activity.

IS THERE A PROSTANOID RELAXANT FACTOR?

In addition to the indomethacin resistant relaxant effects of EpDRF, many studies have demonstrated that interference with the metabolism of arachidonic acid can alter the modulatory role of the epithelium. This suggests that additionally there may be an eicosanoid substance acting as an epithelium derived relaxant factor in the airways. Respiratory epithelial cells can metabolise arachidonic acid by several pathways, the relative importance of each is species dependent (see review by Raeburn, 1990) but one major route of metabolism is by the cyclooxygenase pathway to produce both contractile and relaxant prostanoids.

The role of prostanoids in regulating airway smooth muscle reactivity and the influence of cyclooxygenase inhibitors such as indomethacin on these effects is well established (Orehek et al., 1973, 1975). The influence of the epithelium on these interactions has now become the focus of much interest. Indomethacin treatment of epithelium-containing strips of bronchial and tracheal muscle has been shown to mimic the effects of epithelium removal by augmenting contractile responses to several agents including acetylcholine, methacholine, histamine, LTC_4 and ovalbumin but much diversity is evident (Raeburn, 1990). Indomethacin also has been reported to increase tissue reactivity in the absence of the epithelium (Raeburn, 1990).

Rabbit bronchial preparation produce and release PGE_2 and PGI_2 in an epithelium-dependent manner (Butler et al., 1987). Barnett et al. (1988) have shown that bradykinin releases a smooth muscle relaxant substance from canine epithelial cells in culture. The effect is blocked by indomethacin treatment and, based on this, Barnett et al. (1988) suggest that PGE_2 may be the factor.

Recent studies using radioimmunoassay have demonstrated a reduced release of PGE_2 and PGI_2 in epithelium-denuded compared with intact tissues under basal conditions (Hay et al., 1988a; Folkerts et al., 1989). Following stimulation with muscarinic agonists, histamine or leukotrienes conflicting results have been obtained on prostanoid release from intact and denuded tissues (see Raeburn, 1990).

Possibly the strongest evidence suggesting an epithelium associated prostanoid factor being involved in modulating airway reactivity derives from the studies using exogenously applied arachidonic acid. In epithelium containing tissues arachidonic acid has a relaxant action which is converted to contraction by epithelium removal or pretreatment with indomethacin (Nijkamp & Folkerts, 1987; Farmer et al., 1987a,b; Tschirhart et al., 1987). This relaxant activity of arachidonic acid can be transferred to denuded tissues in bioassay experiments (Farmer et al., 1987b; Tschirhart et al., 1987). An example of this effect is shown in Fig. 3. This suggests that epithelial cyclooxygenase activity normally

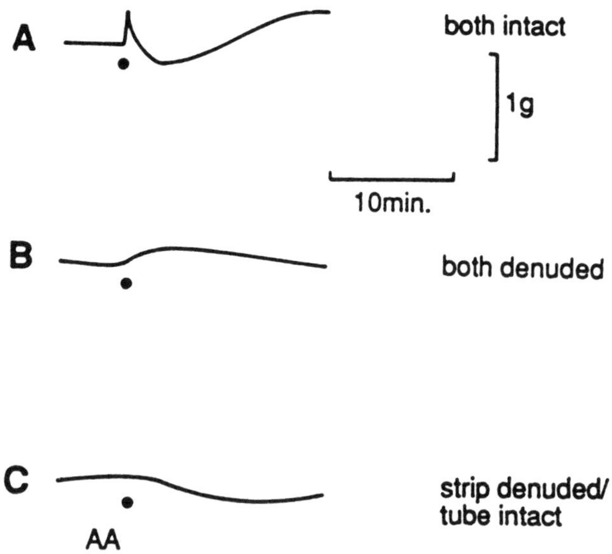

Fig. 3. Responses of coaxial bioassay preparations to arachidonic acid (AA, 0.1 mM) in guinea-pig trachealis. Panel A: donor and acceptor epithelium containing, Panel B: donor and acceptor denuded, Panel C: donor with epithelium and acceptor denuded. Adapted from Farmer (1987b).

metabolizes arachidonic acid to a relaxant prostanoid, the most likely (based on the available evidence) being PGE_2. In the absence of the epithelium no relaxation will be seen. Thus PGE_2 is likely to be a second epithelium-associated relaxant factor.

HOW DOES EpDRF INHIBIT AIRWAY CONTRACTILITY?

As stated previously EpDRF is not a dilator prostanoid nor is it likely to be another metabolite of arachidonic acid (see reviews by Raeburn, 1990; Goldie et al., 1990) but to date no firm candidate has emerged to claim the role. However we do have some understanding of the mechanisms by which EpDRF may be acting.

EpDRF is, on the evidence available, distinct from EDRF and is not nitric oxide. It is unlikely to be acting via stimulation of soluble guanylyl cyclase since it is unaffected by the inhibitor methylene blue. However, Hay et al. (1989), demonstrated an increase in cGMP accompanying epithelium-dependent relaxation to histamine in co-axial bioassay suggesting some stimulation of guanylyl cyclase (possibly particulate?). cAMP production was unaffected. There is now some preliminary data demonstrating an increase in phosphatidylinositol metabolism which accompanies the increased reactivity to some contractile agonists seen on epithelium removal (Hay et al., 1988b) and differential activation of C-kinase may occur in epithelium denuded tissues (Raeburn, 1989).

EpDRF does not act by preventing voltage-dependent Ca^{2+} entry (Raeburn et al., 1987) but may stimulate Na^+/K^+ ATPase activity in the airway smooth muscle to reduce muscle reactivity (Fedan et al., 1988; Raeburn and Fedan, 1989; Lamport and Fedan, 1990). Alternatively, Na^+/K^+ ATPase activity in the epithelium may affect production and release of EpDRF.

From these observations it is probable that EpDRF acts at more than one site to uncouple signal transduction.

EOSINOPHILS AND EPITHELIAL DAMAGE

As discussed earlier, epithelial damage in asthmatic airways is often associated with eosinophil infiltration and the release of cytotoxic eosinophil products such as MBP. A few studies have attempted to replicate these findings in experimental animals. Flavahan et al. (1988) have shown that incubation of epithelium-containing tracheal muscle preparations with purified MBP results in concentration-dependent damage to the epithelium. The damage was accompanied by an increased maximum contractility to histamine and acetylcholine although the tissue sensitivity was not significantly altered. In the absence of the epithelium no effects of MBP were seen. In a similar study (Read et al., 1989) epithelial damage was produced in vitro by Paf-activated eosinophils but not by Paf alone. Non activated eosinophils produced considerably less epithelial damage. In an in vivo preparation, intraepithelial administration of MBP caused an increased reactivity to acetylcholine whereas injection of the muscle was without effect (Brofman et al, 1989). These findings suggest that the release of cytotoxic products from activated eosinophils cause epithelial damage and an increased airway contractility. Flavahan et al. (1988) have suggested that eosinophil-induced epithelial damage can affect EpDRF production and thereby alter airway reactivity.

CONCLUDING COMMENTS

From the data presented it is clear that the epithelium can modulate the reactivity of the underlying airway smooth muscle and this probably is important in the pathophysiology of asthma by contributing to the bronchial hyperreactivity. There is now fairly conclusive evidence that the modulatory effects are due largely to the actions of both prostanoid and non-prostanoid (EpDRF) relaxant factors produced by the epithelium. In some instances altered metabolism and loss of a diffusion barrier may augment the loss of the relaxant factors but the latter effects must be considered minor roles.

REFERENCES

Allegra, L., Fabbri, L.M., Picotti, G., and Mattoli, S. (1989) Bronchial epithelium and asthma, Eur. Resp. J. 2(Suppl. 6), 460s-468s.

Barnett, K., Jacoby, D.B., Nadel, J.A., and Lazarus, S.C. (1988) The effect of epithelial cell supernatant on contractions of isolated canine bronchial smooth muscle, Am. Rev. Resp. Dis. 138, 780-783.

Beasley, R.C., Roberts, J.A., Roche, W.M., and Holgate, S.T. (1988) Bronchial lavage and biopsy findings before and after allergen challenge in mild atopic asthma, Thorax 43, 812P.

Brofman, J.D., White, S.R., Blake, J.S., Munoz, N.M., Gleich, G.J., and Leff, A.R. (1989) Epithelial augmentation of trachealis contraction caused by major basic protein of eosinophils, J. Appl. Physiol. 66, 1867-1873.

Butler, G.B., Adler, K.B., Evans, J.N., Morgan, D.W., and Szarek, J.L. (1987) Modulation of rabbit airway smooth muscle responsiveness by respiratory epithelium, Am. Rev. Resp. Dis. 135, 1099-1104.

Dunnill, M.S. (1960) The pathology of asthma, with special reference to changes in the bronchial mucosa, J. Clin. Pathol. 13, 27-33.

Elia, C., Bucca, C., Rolla, G., Scappaticci, E., and Cantino, D. (1988) A freeze-fracture study of human bronchial epithelium in normal, bronchitic and asthmatic subjects, J. Submicrosc. Cytol. Pathol. 20, 509-517.

Farmer, S.G., Hay, D.W.P., Raeburn, D., and Fedan, J.S. (1987a) Relaxation of guinea pig tracheal smooth muscle to arachidonate is converted to contraction following epithelium removal, Br. J. Pharmacol. 92, 231-236.

Farmer, S.G., Hay, D.W.P., Raeburn, D., and Fedan, J.S. (1987b) Influence of the epithelium on airway responses to bronchorelaxant drugs: is there an epithelium-derived factor? In: International seminar on relaxant factors: Their significance in cardiovascular and respiratory diseases, London, July 1987.

Fedan, J.S., Hay, D.W.P., Farmer, S.G., and Raeburn, D. (1988) Epithelial cells: Modulation of airway smooth muscle reactivity. In: Asthma: Basic mechanisms and clinical management (I.W. Rodger, P.J. Barnes and N.C. Thomson, Eds), Academic Press, New York, pp. 143-162.

Fernandes, L.B., Paterson, J.W., and Goldie, R.G. (1989) Co-axial bioassay of a smooth muscle relaxant factor released from guinea-pig tracheal epithelium, Br. J. Pharmacol. 96, 117-124.

Filley, W.V., Holley, K.E., Kephart, G.M., and Gleich, G.J. (1982) Identification by immunofluorescence of eosinophil granule major basic protein in lung tissues of patients with bronchial asthma, Lancet II, 11-16.

Flavahan, N.A., and Vanhoutte, P.M. (1985) The respiratory epithelium releases a smooth muscle relaxing factor, Chest 87 (suppl.), 189S-190S.

Flavahan, N.A., Aarhus, L.L., Rimele, T.J., and Vanhoutte, P.M. (1985) Respiratory epithelium inhibits bronchial smooth muscle tone, J. Appl. Physiol. 58, 834-838.
Flavahan, N.A., Slifman, N.R., Gleich, G.J., and Vanhoutte, P.M. (1988) Human eosinophil major basic protein causes hyperreactivity of respiratory smooth muscle, Am. Rev. Resp. Dis. 138, 685-688.
Folkerts, G., Engels, F., and Nijkamp, F.P. (1989) Respiratory airway hyperreactivity coincides with decreased epithelium-derived PGE_2, Agents Actions 26, 68-69.
Furchgott, R.F. (1984) The role of endothelium in the responses of vascular smooth muscle to drugs, Ann. Rev. Pharmacol. Toxicol. 24, 175-197.
Goldie, R.G., Fernandes, L.B., Farmer, S.G., and Hay, D.W.P. (1990) Airway epithelium-derived inhibitory factor, Trends Pharmacol. Sci. 11, 67-70.
Guc, M.O., Ilhan, M., and Kayaalp, S.O. (1988) The rat anococcygeus muscle is a convenient bioassay organ for the airway epithelium-derived relaxant factor, Eur. J. Pharmacol. 148, 405-409.
Hay, D.W.P., Raeburn, D., Farmer, S.G., Fleming, W.W., and Fedan, J.S. (1986) Epithelium modulates the reactivity of ovalbumin-sensitized guinea-pig airway smooth muscle, Life Sci. 38, 2461-2468.
Hay, D.W.P., Muccitelli, R.M., Horstemeyer, D.L., Wilson, K.A., and Raeburn, D. (1987) Demonstration of the release of an epithelium-derived inhibitory factor from a novel preparation of guinea-pig trachea, Eur. J. Pharmacol. 129, 247-250.
Hay, D.W.P., Muccitelli, R.M., Horstemeyer, D.L., and Raeburn, D. (1988a) Is the epithelium-derived inhibitory factor in guinea-pig trachea a prostanoid?, Prostaglandins 35, 625-637.
Hay, D.W.P., Muccitelli, R.M., and Raeburn, D. (1988b) Does the epithelium-derived inhibitory factor (EpDIF) act via inhibition of phosphatidylinositol (PI) turnover in guinea-pig trachea (GPT)?, FASEB. J. 2, A1057.
Hay, D.W.P., Fard, A., and Muccitelli, R.M. (1989) Correlation between the relaxation of rat aorta induced by the airway epithelium-derived inhibitory factor and cyclic nucleotide levels, Am. Rev. Resp. Dis. 139, A352.
Holroyde, M.C. (1986) The influence of epithelium on the responsiveness of guinea-pig isolated trachea, Br. J. Pharmacol. 87, 501-507.
Ilhan, M., and Sahin, I. (1986) Tracheal epithelium releases a vascular smooth muscle relaxant factor: Demonstration by bioassay, Eur. J. Pharmacol. 131, 293-296.
Jeffery, P.K., Wardlaw, A.J., Nelson, F.C., Collins, J.V., and Kay, A.B. (1989) Bronchial biopsies in asthma: An ultrastructural, quantitative study and correlation with hyperreactivity, Am. Rev. Resp. Dis. 140, 1745-1753.
Laitinen, L.A., Heino, M., Laitinen, A., Kava, T., and Haahtela, T. (1985) Damage of the airway epithelium and bronchial reactivity in patients with asthma, Am. Rev. Resp. Dis. 131, 599-606.

Lamport, S.J., and Fedan, J.S. (1990) Modulation of the reactivity of the guinea-pig isolated trachealis by respiratory epithelium: Effects of cooling, Br. J. Pharmacol. 99, 369-373.
Lozewicz, S., Wells, C., Gomez, E., Ferguson, H., Richman, P., Devalia, J., and Davies, R.J. (1990) Morphological integrity of the bronchial epithelium in mild asthma, Thorax 45, 12-15
Naline, E., Devillier, P., Drapeau, G., Toty, L., Backdach, H., Regoli, D., and Advenier, C. (1989) Characterization of neurokinin effects and receptor selectivity in human isolated bronchus, Am. Rev. Resp. Dis. 140, 679-686.
Nijkamp, F.P., and Folkerts, G. (1987) Reversal of arachidonic-acid induced guinea-pig tracheal relaxation into contraction after epithelium removal, Eur. J. Pharmacol. 131, 315-316.
Orehek, J., Douglas, J.S., Lewis, A.J., and Bouhuys, A. (1973) Prostaglandin regulation of airway smooth muscle tone. Nature (New Biol.) 245, 84-85.
Orehek, J., Douglas, J.S., and Bouhuys, A. (1975) Contractile responses of the guinea-pig trachea in vitro: Modification by prostaglandin synthesis-inhibiting drugs, J. Pharmacol. Exp. Ther. 194, 554-564.
Raeburn, D., Hay, D.W.P., and Fedan, J.S. (1987) Calcium uptake into guinea-pig trachealis: The effect of epithelium removal, Cell Calcium 8, 429-436.
Raeburn, D. (1989) Do phorbol esters produce relaxation of tracheal muscle by generation of arachidonic acid from airway epithelium?, Br. J. Pharmacol. 98, 785P.
Raeburn, D., and Fedan, J.S. (1989) The effects of alterations in electrogenic Na+/K+ pumping in guinea-pig isolated trachealis: Their modulation by the epithelium, Br. J. Pharmacol. 98, 343-350.
Raeburn, D. (1990) Eicosanoids, epithelium and airway reactivity, Gen. Pharmacol. 21, 11-16.
Read, R.C., Yukawa, T., Kroegel, C., Chung, K.F., Rutman, A., Wilson, R., Cole, P.J., and Barnes, P.J. (1989) In vitro interaction of activated eosinophils and neutrophils with guinea pig airway epithelium, Thorax 44, 896P.
Sanerkin, N.G., and Evans, D.M.D. (1965) The sputum in bronchial asthma: pathogonomic patterns, J. Path. Bact. 89, 535-541.
Tschirhart, E., Frossard, N., Bertrand, C., and Landry, Y. (1987) Arachidonic acid metabolites and airway epithelium dependent relaxant factor, J. Pharmacol. Exp. Ther. 243, 310-316.
Undem, B.J., Raible, D.J., Adkinson, N.F., and Adams, G.K. (1987) Effect of removal of epithelium on antigen-induced smooth muscle contraction and mediator release from guinea pig isolated trachea, J. Pharmacol. Exp. Ther. 244, 659-665.
Vanhoutte, P.M. (1987) Airway epithelium and bronchial reactivity, Can. J. Physiol. Pharmacol. 65, 448-450.
Vanhoutte, P.M. (1988) Epithelium-derived relaxing factor(s) and bronchial reactivity, Am. Rev. Resp. Dis. 138, S24-S30.

AAS 31:
Mediators in
Airway Hyperreactivity

THE ROLE OF EPITHELIUM IN THE RESPONSIVENESS OF THE BRONCHI TO STIMULI

H.W. Mitchell, K.E. Willet and M.P. Sparrow

Physiology Dept, University of Western Australia, Nedlands 6009, Australia

SUMMARY: Airway narrowing in response to different modes of stimuli was measured using a perfused bronchial segment. Acetylcholine, carbachol, histamine, high $[K^+]$ and vanadate perfused through the lumen gave small responses as shown by the reduction in flow, but fully constricted the airway when applied to the outside. ACh was 29 times more sensitive on the outside. When the epithelium was removed airway narrowing by these stimuli was increased to equal that on the outside. It was concluded that the role of the epithelia as a barrier is all important. Evidence for an EpDIF released by the epithelium could not be obtained.

The epithelium lining the airways of the lung may function as a permeability barrier (Holroyde, 1986), by actively protecting the smooth muscle by elaborating an epithelial-derived inhibitory factor (EpDIF) (Flavahan *et al.*,1985; Goldie *et al.*,1986) and as an uptake and metabolic role for many substances (Farmer *et al.*, 1987). Although EpDIF can be demonstrated *in vitro* its physiological significance remains uncertain (Goldie *et al.*, 1990). Likewise the barrier properties of the epithelium remain controversial. This is largely because of the use of isolated strips of airway wall where neither EpDIF production nor a diffusion barrier can be unequivocally assessed.

Airway narrowing is the parameter of physiological significance and can be measured using intact bronchial segments (Mitchell *et al.*, 1989). With this preparation we have shown using several modes of stimulation that a major function of the epithelium is that of a barrier preventing the penetration of substances from the lumen.

RESULTS

Airway narrowing responses of perfused segments depended on the surface of the tissue to which the stimulating agent was presented. Figure 1 shows that the sensitivity (EC_{50}) of the bronchial segments to ACh was increased 29 fold from 69μM perfused through the lumen to 2.4μM to the outside (P<0.01). This difference in sensitivity between the inside and the outside was more striking using carbachol, histamine, K^+ depolarising solution, KCl or vanadate (Fig. 2).

Fig 1

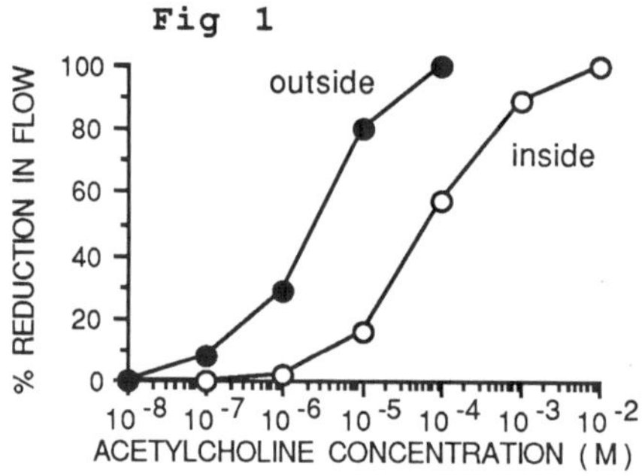

Fig 2

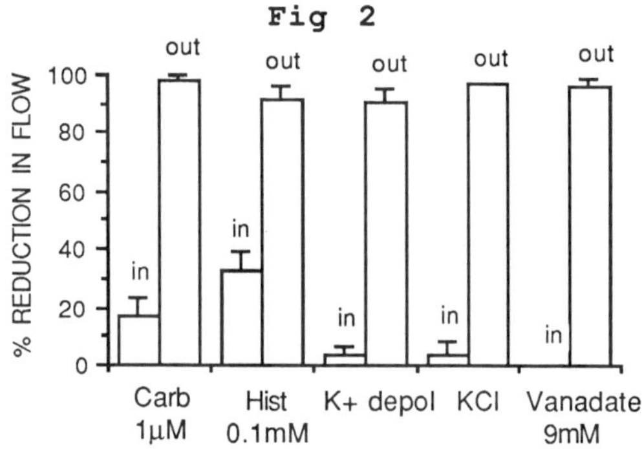

Fig. 1. Bronchial segments 20mm long with an external diameter of 3mm at the distal end were dissected from fresh pig lungs and perfused with Krebs at $5cmH_2O$ (Mitchell *et al.*, 1989) which gave a resting flow rate of 33ml/min. Narrowing is shown as a % reduction in flow. ACh was added to the perfusate (○ inside) or to the Krebs solution bathing the outside (● outside). Points are mean responses (n=4 pigs).

Fig. 2. Agents exposed to the inside and outside of the segment. Mean±SE of 3-6 pigs. K^+ depolarising solution was 80mM K_2SO_4 replacing NaCl in Krebs. KCl solution contained 121mM KCl in place of NaCl. Vanadate (VO_3^-) solution was 9mM ammonium vanadate in Krebs.

The results suggested that the epithelial layer was acting as a barrier, reducing or preventing the diffusion of these agents to the smooth muscle. Fig. 3 shows that the ACh sensitivity of segments from which the epithelium had been stripped was increased 37 fold, the EC_{50} shifting from 60.3μM to 1.6μM ($P<0.01$, n=6 pigs) and was now comparable with that seen outside (EC_{50} 2.4μM). Likewise perfusion of carbachol 1μM, K^+ depolarising solution, KCl solution or 9mM VO_3^- through the lumen now produced complete or near complete abolition of flow.

If an EpDIF was elaborated by the epithelium it would have to diffuse across the submucosa to inhibit smooth muscle contraction. But smooth muscle contraction was not suppressed when any of the above agents were added to the outside even when that agent continued to be perfused through the inside (Fig. 4).

Fig 3

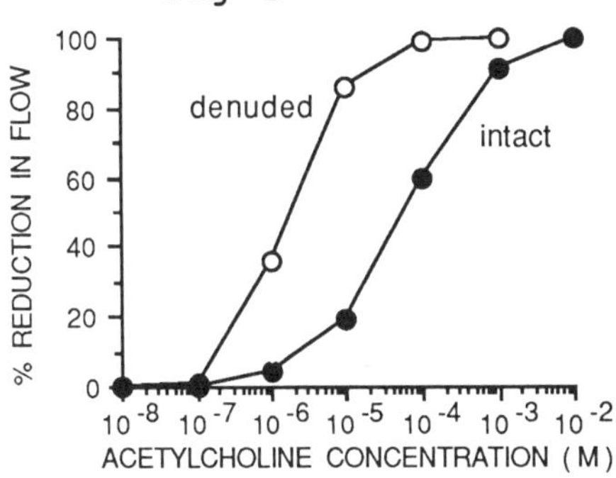

Fig 4

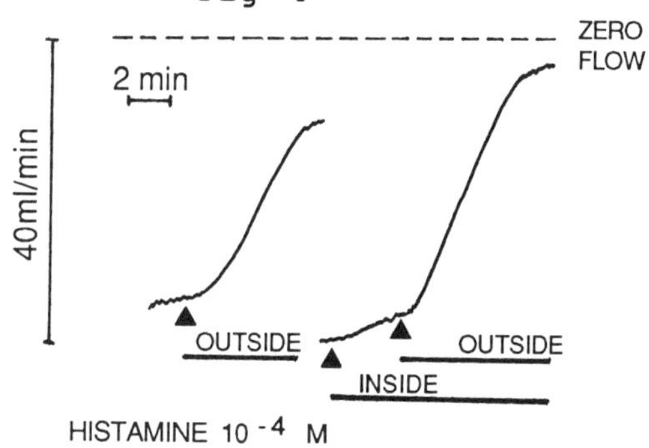

DISCUSSION

We have demonstrated here that the epithelium lining the bronchi in pig lungs is an effective barrier to solute molecules. Perfused carbachol 1μM, ACh 10μM, histamine 0.1mM, K^+ depolarising solution, KCl and vanadate had small or negligible effects on flow whereas on the outside they caused near cessation of flow. After removal of the epithelium the effect of these agents on the inside was virtually the same as that applied to the outside. Other workers use strips of airway wall, where an epithelial surface, a serosal surface and cut edges are exposed to the bathing fluid. This is possibly why relatively small shifts of 2-5 fold are seen (Goldie *et el.*, 1986; Flavahan et al., 1985) compared with the 30-40 fold shifts reported here. Our preparation, an intact tube, completely isolates the mucosa from the outside of the airway. Furthermore smooth muscle contraction was not suppressed when stimulated from the outside (Fig 4) showing that an EpDIF, if produced, was not having any effect. It is well known that the epithelial cells lining tubular organs function as a barrier with the tight junctions between the cells varying greatly in their capacity to hinder the penetration of molecules. The results described here provide a dramatic demonstration of the effectiveness of this barrier in the airways and show that it is of major importance in airway narrowing and bronchial responsiveness.

REFERENCES

Farmer, S.G., Hay, D.W.P., Raeburn, D. and Fedan, J.S. (1987), Relaxation of guinea-pig tracheal smooth muscle to arachidonate is converted to contraction following epithelium removal. Br. J. Pharmac. 92, 231-236.

Flavahan, N.A., Aarhus, L.L., Rimele, T.J. and Vanhoutte, P.M. (1985), Respiratory epithelium inhibits bronchial smooth muscle tone. J. Appl. Physiol. 58, 834-838.

Goldie, R.G., Papadimitriou, J.M., Paterson, J.W., Rigby, P.J. Self, H.M. and Spina, D.(1986), Influence of the epithelium on responsiveness of guinea-pig isolated trachea to contractile and relaxant agonists. Br. J. Pharmac. 87, 5-14.

Goldie, R.G., Fernandes, L.B., Farmer, S.G. and Hay, D.W.P. (1990), Airway epithelium-derived inhibitory factor. TIPS 11, 67-70.

Holroyde, M.C. (1986), The influence of epithelium on the responsiveness of guinea-pig isolated trachea. Br. J. Pharmac. 87, 501-507.

Mitchell, H.W., Willet, K.W. and Sparrow, M.P. (1989), Perfused segment and bronchial strip: narrowing vs isometric force by mediators. J. Appl. Physiol. 66, 2704-2709.

AAS 31:
Mediators in
Airway Hyperreactivity

ADDITIVE EFFECT OF EPITHELIAL DENUDATION AND LOW LEVELS OF INFLAMMATORY MEDIATORS ON THE SENSITIVITY OF ISOLATED HUMAN AIRWAYS TO METHACHOLINE

R.C. Jongejan, J.C. de Jongste, H.C. Raatgeep, I.L. Bonta and K.F. Kerrebijn

Department of Pediatrics, Subdivision of Pediatric Respiratory Medicine, and Department of Pharmacology, Erasmus University / Sophia Children's Hospital, 3038 GE Rotterdam, The Netherlands.

SUMMARY: The presence of low concentrations of histamine or the stable thromboxane analogue U46619 and the removal of the epithelium separately and addictively increase the sensitivity of isolated human airways to methacholine. This raises the possibility that these factors play a role in the pathogenesis of bronchial hyperresponsiveness to inhaled methacholine in asthma.

In bronchial biopsies from clinically stable allergic asthmatics epithelial damage has been observed (Laitinen et al., 1985). In this type of patients both the number of epithelial cells and the amount of inflammatory mediators such as histamine and thromboxane A_2 (TxA_2) that are present in the bronchoalveolar lavage fluid are related to the airway responsiveness to inhaled methacholine (Beasley et al., 1989, Gravelyn et al., 1988). These findings suggest that in asthma epithelial damage and the ongoing production of inflammatory mediators in quantities which do not lead to bronchoconstriction both contribute to bronchial hyperresponsiveness. Indeed, epithelial denudation has been found to increase the responsiveness of isolated non-asthmatic human airways to acetylcholine (Aizawa et al., 1988), and we have shown that the presence of threshold concentrations of

twofold increase in sensitivity of isolated human airways to methacholine (Jongejan et al., 1990). To clarify if the increase in smooth muscle responsiveness caused by low levels of inflammatory mediators adds to the increased responsiveness caused by the absence of epithelium we investigated the effect of low levels of inflammatory mediators on the cholinergic responsiveness of isolated human airways with and without epithelium.

MATERIALS AND METHODS

Human lung tissue was obtained at thoracotomies. Non-cartilaginous bronchi (Ø 1-2 mm) were identified, cannulated and cleaned from adherent tissue (Jongejan et al., 1988). Each bronchial tube was cut into two adjacent segments which were cut open into strips. In one of each pair of strips the luminal side was gently rubbed with a wet gauze to remove the epithelium. The strips were stored overnight in a slow flow of cold Krebs-Henseleit buffer. The following day the preparations were mounted in organ baths of 10 ml between a hook at the bottom of the bath and the arm of an isotonic transducer which was loaded with a weight of 250 mg. First, all preparations were contracted with methacholine (10^{-5}M, 10^{-4}M) twice. Next on each pair of strips a cumulative concentration response curve (CCRC) to methacholine (10^{-8}M - 10^{-4}M) was obtained followed by washing. Then a threshold dose of histamine (10^{-8}M) or U46619 (10^{-9}M) was added to both strips. Fifteen minutes later a second CCRC to methacholine was obtained in the presence of the mediator and a third CCRC after washout. Parallel control experiments were done where the second of the three consecutive CCRC was made after precontraction with a threshold concentration of methacholine (3×10^{-7}M). Removal of the epithelium was confirmed histologically. The results were analyzed with repeated measurements analysis of variance (ANOVA, $\alpha=0.05$).

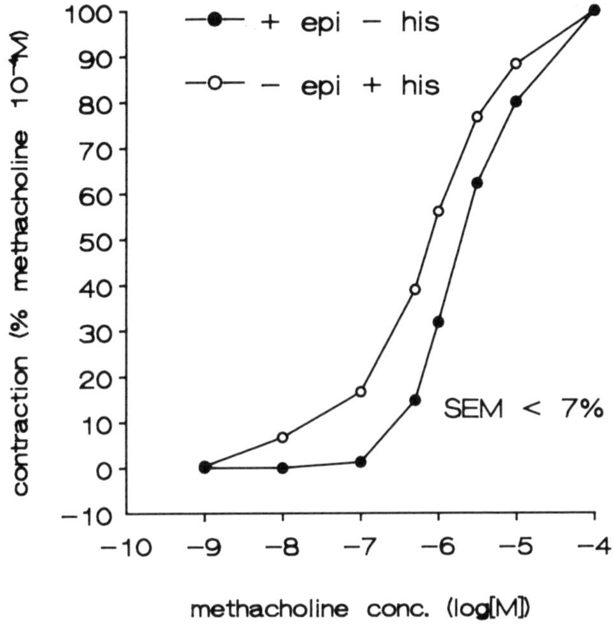

Figure 1. Mean CCRC to methacholine in strips <u>with</u> epithelium in the <u>absence</u> of histamine (10^{-8} M) (open symbols) and strips <u>without</u> epithelium in the <u>presence</u> of histamine (10^{-8} M) (closed symbols).

RESULTS

In the absence of epithelium and presence of histamine the mean CCRC was shifted leftwards (Fig. 1). For U46619 the results were similar. Analysis of variance showed that both the absence of epithelium and the presence of either histamine or U46619 caused a significant leftward shift of the dose response curve to methacholine ($P<0.05$).

DISCUSSION

Our data indicate that the presence of low concentrations of histamine or thromboxane A_2 and the absence of epithelium separately and addictively increase the sensitivity of human airway smooth muscle to methacholine. In vivo studies indicate that low concentrations of histamine and thromboxane A_2 as well as damage of epithelium can both be found in the airways of symptom free asthmatics with hyperreactivity to inhaled methacholine. Therefore our data suggest that these factors may both contribute independently to an increased responsiveness of the airway muscle to inhaled methacholine in bronchial asthma. However, these results can not explain the 10 - 1000 fold increase in sensitivity to inhaled methacholine which is often seen in asthmatics in vivo. Therefore additional factors must also play a role in asthmatic bronchial hyperreactivity to inhaled methacholine.

Acknowledgements: The authors thank the Departments of Pathology, Pulmonology and Thoracic Surgery of the Ikazia and Leyenburg Hospitals, the Zuiderziekenhuis and the University Hospital of the Erasmus University for providing the lung tissue.
Supported by a grant of the Netherlands Asthma Foundation.

REFERENCES

Aizawa, H., Miyazaki, N., Shigematsu N., and Tomooka M. (1988) A possible role of airway epithelium in modulating hyperresponsiveness. Br. J. Pharmacol. 93, 139-145.

Beasley, R., Roche, P.D., Roberts, J.A., and Holgate, S.T. (1989) Cellular events in the bronchi in mild asthma and after bronchial provocation. Am. Rev. Respir. Dis. 139, 806-817.

Gravelyn, T.R., Pan, P.M., and Eschenbacher, W.L. (1988) Mediator release in an isolated airway segment in subjects with asthma. Am. Rev. Respir. Dis. 137, 641-646.

Jongejan, R.C., De Jongste, J.C., Van Strik, R., Raatgeep, R.C., Bonta., I.W., and Kerrebijn, K.F. (1989) Measurement of human small airway smooth muscle function in vitro, comparison of bronchiolar strips and segments. J. Pharmacol. Meth. 20, 135-142.

Jongejan, R.C., De Jongste, J.C., Raatgeep, R.C., Bonta, I.L., and Kerrebijn, K.F. (1990) Effects of inflammatory mediators on the responsiveness of isolated human airways to methacholine. Am. Rev. Respir. Dis., in press.

Laitinen, L.A., Heino, M., Laitinen, A., Kava T., Haahtela T. (1985) Damage of the epithelium and bronchial reactivity in patients with asthma. Am. Rev. Respir. Dis. 131, 599-606.

AAS 31:
Mediators in
Airway Hyperreactivity

EPITHELIUM-DERIVED LINOLEIC ACID METABOLITES MODULATE AIRWAY SMOOTH MUSCLE FUNCTION.

Paul A.J. Henricks, Ferdi Engels, Betty van Esch, Henk J. van der Linde, Moira J. Oosthuizen and Frans P. Nijkamp.

Department of Pharmacology, Faculty of Pharmacy, University of Utrecht, Catharijnesingel 60, 3511 GH Utrecht, The Netherlands.

SUMMARY: Cultured epithelial cells obtained from guinea pig tracheal preparations metabolized arachidonic acid into 5- and 15-hydroxy-eicosatetraenoic acid and into the prostaglandins E_2 and $F_{2\alpha}$. Linoleic acid was converted by the epithelial cells into 9-hydroxy-octadecadienoic acid (9-HODE) and smaller amounts of 13-HODE. It was further investigated whether linoleic acid metabolites are of importance for the regulation of airway smooth muscle function. 13-HODE caused an increase of maximal contraction of tracheal rings to histamine, while 9-HODE had no effect.

Airway epithelial cells play an important role in airway function. Damage of the epithelial lining is associated with airway smooth muscle hyperreactivity for contractile agents (Vanhoutte, 1988). Production of fatty acid derived mediators may be one of the mechanisms by which epithelial cells modulate airway smooth muscle function. Most of the research concerning the production and the biological activity of fatty acid metabolites has been directed towards arachidonic acid metabolism and metabolites (Eling et al., 1988), whereas little attention has been paid to the metabolism and metabolites of linoleic acid. In this study it was investigated which fatty acid metabolites can be formed by cultured guinea pig tracheal epithelial cells and whether linoleic acid metabolites are able to influence the reactivity of airway smooth muscle function.

MATERIALS AND METHODS

Epithelial cells were obtained from guinea pig tracheas by incubation with pronase E for 18h at 4°C (Wu et al., 1985). Cells were suspended in 3.5 ml supplemented Ham F12 medium and placed in 35 mm cell culture dishes. The dishes were incubated at 37°C in a humidified atmosphere of 5% CO_2 in air.

The epithelial cell cultures were incubated with exogenous $[^{14}C]$arachidonic acid or with $[^{14}C]$linoleic acid for 15 min at 37°C after 7 days of culture. Incubation fluids were analyzed by reverse-phase high performance liquid chromatography (Oosthuizen et al., 1990).

Guinea pig tracheas were cut into rings, which were placed in organ baths and connected to isometric transducers. A dose-response curve to cumulative concentrations of histamine was performed after a 30 min incubation with 10 µM 9- or 13-HODE.

RESULTS

The epithelial cell cultures contained 95% epithelial cells after 7 days of culturing as determined by an indirect immunoperoxidase technique using monoclonal antibodies directed against cytokeratins.

Incubation of the cultured epithelial cells for 15 min in the presence of exogenous radiolabeled arachidonic acid mainly led to the formation of 5- and 15-hydroxyeicosatetraenoic acid (5- and 15-HETE) and the prostaglandins (PG) E_2 and $F_{2\alpha}$ (Table I). 9-HODE and 13-HODE were detected after incubation of the cultured epithelial cells with exogenous radiolabeled linoleic acid (Table I).

An increased response to cumulative concentrations of histamine was observed when tracheal preparations were incubated with 10 µM 13-HODE for 30 min as compared to control incubations (1642 ± 119 mgf vs 1044 ± 327 mgf). No effects on the contraction of the tracheal preparations was detected when the preparations had been incubated with 9-HODE.

Tabel I. Production of fatty acid metabolites by primary cultures of guinea pig tracheal epithelial cells.

5-HETE	26 ± 7 pmol/well
15-HETE	29 ± 7 pmol/well
$PGF_{2\alpha}$	37 ± 8 pmol/well
PGE_2	32 ± 4 pmol/well
9-HODE	319 ± 54 pmol/well
13-HODE	53 ± 18 pmol/well

DISCUSSION

Considerable differences in arachidonic acid metabolism by respiratory epithelial cells from different animal species have been observed (Eling et al., 1988). Recently we have found that freshly isolated tracheal epithelial cells from guinea pigs metabolize arachidonic acid and linoleic acid into their mono-hydroxy-derivatives (Oosthuizen et al., 1990). The present results confirm these findings and also show that cultured cells are capable to produce PGE_2 and $PGF_{2\alpha}$ in contrast to freshly isolated guinea pig tracheal epithelial cells. Also isolated rabbit and rat tracheal epithelial cells only develop the ability to metabolize arachidonic acid into prostaglandins under culture conditions (Eling et al., 1988).

A lot of research has been carried out concerning the biological activity of arachidonic acid metabolites with respect to lung function. In contrast, less is known about the linoleic acid metabolites. 9- and 13-HODE interfere with reactive oxygen species released by pulmonary alveolar macrophages (Engels et al., 1989) and possess chemotactic activity for polymorphonuclear cells (Henricks et al., 1990). In this paper we demonstrate that incubation of tracheal segments with 13-HODE induced an increased contractile response to histamine. Further investigations in our laboratory have shown that 13-HODE also modulated the response of airway smooth muscle to other contractile agents (Engels et al., 1990).

Acknowledgements: This study was supported financially by the Dutch Asthma Foundation (grant 86.17).

REFERENCES

Eling, T.E., Henke, D., and Danilowicz, R. (1988) Arachidonic acid metabolism in respiratory epithelial cells. Gen. Pharmacol. 19, 313-316.

Engels, F., Henricks, P.A.J., Van der Linde, H.J. and Nijkamp, F.P. (1990) Modulation of guinea pig airway reactivity by the linoleic acid metabolite 13-hydroxy-octadecadienoic acid (13-HODE). In: Mediators in Airway Hyperreactivity (F.P. Nijkamp, F. Engels, P.A.J. Henricks and A.J.M. van Oosterhout, Eds), Agents Actions Supplements, Birkhäuser Verlag, Basel, this issue, pp. 113-117.

Engels, F., Henricks, P.A.J., Van der Vliet, H. and Nijkamp, F.P. (1989) Modulatory activity of 9-hydroxy- and 9-hydroperoxy-octadecadienoic acid towards reactive oxygen species from guinea-pig pulmonary macrophages. Eur. J. Biochem. 184, 197-203.

Henricks, P.A.J., Engels, E., Van der Vliet, H., and Nijkamp F.P. (1990) 9- and 13-hydroxy-linoleic acid possess chemotactic activity for bovine and human polymorphonuclear leukocytes, submitted.

Oosthuizen, M.J., Engels, F., Van Esch, B., Henricks, P.A.J., and Nijkamp, F.P. (1990) Production of arachidonic and linoleic acid metabolites by guinea pig tracheal epithelial cells. Inflammation 14, 401-408.

Vanhoutte, P.M. (1988) Epithelium-derived relaxing factor(s) and bronchial reactivity. Am. Rev. Respir. Dis. 138, S24-S30.

Wu, R., Yankaskas, J., Cheng, E., Knowles, M.R., and Boucher, R. (1985) Growth and differentiation of human nasal epithelial cells in culture. Am. Rev. Respir. Dis. 132, 311-320.

AUTHOR INDEX

SUBJECT INDEX

AGENTS AND ACTIONS SUPPLEMENTS

Edited by K.Brune

AAS 25
Non-Opioid (OTC)
Analgesics - Risks/Benefits in Perspective
Edited by K.Brune.
ISBN 3-7643-2251-9

AAS 26
Cologne Artherosclerosis Conference
No 4: Cholesterol-Homeostasis
Edited by M.J. Parnham, R. Niemann.
ISBN 3-7643-2247-0

AAS 27
Anti-Inflammatory Drugs from Plant and Marine Sources
Edited by D.A. Lewis.
ISBN 3-7643-2265-9

AAS 28
Intrinsic Asthma
Edited by M.Schmitz-Schumann, G. Menz, U. Costable, C.P. Page.
ISBN 3-7643-2289-6

AAS 29
Risk Factors for Adverse Drug Reactions - Epidemiological Approaches
Edited by E. Weber, D.H. Lawson, R. Hoigné.
ISBN 3-7643-2372-8

AAS 30
Inflammatory Indices in Chronic Bronchitis
Edited by C.G.A. Persson, R. Brattsand, L.A. Laitinen, P. Venge.
ISBN 3-7643-2370-1

New Series
ADVANCES IN PHARMACOLOGICAL SCIENES

APS
Effects of Nicotine on Biological Systems
Edited by F. Adelkofer, K. Thurau.
ISBN 3-7643-2519-4

APS
Animal Models in Psycho-pharmacology
Edited by B. Olivier, J. Mos, J.L. Slangen.
ISBN 3-7643-2503-8

APS
The Pharmacology of Adrenoreceptors: Structure, Mechanisms, Function
Edited by E. Szabadi, C.-M. Bradshaw.
ISBN 3-7643-2518-6